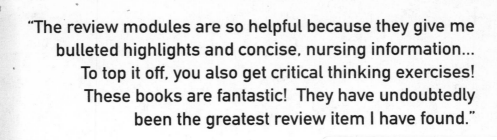

"The review modules are so helpful because they give me bulleted highlights and concise, nursing information... To top it off, you also get critical thinking exercises! These books are fantastic! They have undoubtedly been the greatest review item I have found."

Terim Richards *Nursing student*

"I immediately went to my nurse manager after I failed the NCLEX® and she referred me to ATI. I was able to discover the areas I was weak in, and focused on those areas in the review modules and online assessments. I was much more prepared the second time around!"

Molly Obetz *Nursing student*

"The ATI review books were very helpful in preparing me for the NCLEX®. I really utilized the review summaries and the critical thinking exercises at the end of each chapter. It was nice to review the key points in the areas I was weak in and not have to read the entire book."

Lindsey Koeble *Nursing student*

"I attribute my success totally to ATI. That is the one thing I used between my first and second attempt at the NCLEX®....with ATI I passed!"

Danielle Platt *Nurse Manager • Children's Mercy Hospital • Kansas City, MO*

"The year our hospital did not use the ATI program, we experienced a 15% decrease in the NCLEX® pass rates. We reinstated the ATI program the following year and had a 90% success rate."

"As a manager, I have witnessed graduate nurses fail the NCLEX® and the devastating effects it has on their morale. Once the nurses started using ATI, it was amazing to see the confidence they had in themselves and their ability to go forward and take the NCLEX® exam."

Mary Moss *Associate Dean of Nursing and Health Programs • Mid-State Technical College • Rapids, WI*

"I like that ATI lets students know what to expect from the NCLEX®, helps them plan their study time and tells them what to do in the days and weeks before the exam. It is different from most of the NCLEX® review books on the market."

Nursing Leadership and Management
Review Module Edition 3.0

Contributors

Anita W. Finkelman, RN, MSN

Adjunct Associate Professor, Clinical Nursing
College of Nursing, University of Cincinnati
Cincinnati, Ohio
President, Resources for Excellence
Textbook Author

Patricia A. Jamerson, RNC, PhD

Professor of Nursing
Barnes College of Nursing, University of Missouri
St. Louis, Missouri
Textbook Author

Joan Luckmann, RN, MA

University of Washington
Seattle, Washington
Textbook Author

Penny Marshall-Chura, PhD, MSN

Professor of Nursing
Assistant Dean
Johnson County Community College
Overland Park, Kansas

Peggy Monahan, RN, PhD, MSN

Associate Professor of Nursing
Marian College
Fond du Lac, Wisconsin

Lynn C. Parsons, RN, DSN

Professor of Nursing
Associate Dean
College of Basic and Applied Sciences
Middle Tennessee State University
Murfreeboro, Tennessee

Editor-in-Chief

Leslie Schaaf Treas, RN, PhD(c), MSN, CNNP

Director of Research and Development
Assessment Technologies Institute™, LLC
Overland Park, Kansas

Editors

Jim Hauschildt, RN, EdD, MA

Director of Product Development
Assessment Technologies Institute™, LLC
Overland Park, Kansas

Jennifer Bush, BA, MS

Associate Editor
Assessment Technologies Institute™, LLC
Overland Park, Kansas

Copyright Notice

Important Notice to the Reader of this Publication

Assessment Technologies Institute™, LLC is the publisher of this publication. The publisher reserves the right to modify, change, or update the content of this publication at any time. The content of this publication, such as text, graphics, images, information obtained from the publisher's licensors, and other material contained in this publication are for informational purposes only. The content is not providing medical advice, and is not intended to be a substitute for professional medical advice, diagnosis, or treatment.

Always seek the advice of your primary care provider or other qualified health provider with any questions you may have regarding a medical condition. Never disregard professional medical advice or delay in seeking it because of something you have read in this publication. If you think you may have a medical emergency, call your primary care provider or 911 immediately.

The publisher does not recommend or endorse any specific tests, primary care providers, products, procedures, processes, opinions, or other information that may be mentioned in this publication. Reliance on any information provided by the publisher, the publisher's employees, or others contributing to the content at the invitation of the publisher, is solely at your own risk. Healthcare professionals need to use their own clinical judgment in interpreting the content of this publication, and details such as medications, dosages or laboratory tests and results should always be confirmed with other resources.†

This publication may contain health or medical-related materials that are sexually explicit. If you find these materials offensive, you may not want to use this publication.

The publishers, editors, advisors, and reviewers make no representations or warranties of any kind or nature, including, but not limited to, the accuracy, reliability, completeness, currentness, timeliness, or the warranties of fitness for a particular purpose or merchantability, nor are any such representations implied with respect to the content herein (with such content to include text and graphics), and the publishers, editors, advisors, and reviewers take no responsibility with respect to such content. The publishers, editors, advisors, and reviewers shall not be liable for any actual, incidental, special, consequential, punitive or exemplary damages (or any other type of damages) resulting, in whole or in part, from the reader's use of, or reliance upon, such content.

Introduction to Assessment–Driven Review

To prepare candidates for the licensure exam, many different methods have been used. Assessment Technologies Institute™, LLC, (ATI) offers Assessment–Driven Review™ (ADR), a newer approach for customized board review based on candidate performance on a series of content-based assessments.

The ADR method is a four-part process that serves as a type of competency-assessment for preparation for the NCLEX-RN®. The goal is to increase preparedness and subsequent pass rate on the licensure exam. Used as a comprehensive program, the ADR is designed to help learners focus their review and remediation efforts, thereby increasing their confidence and familiarity with the NCLEX-RN® content. This type of program identifies learners at risk for failure in the early stages of nursing education and provides a path for prescriptive learning prior to the licensure examination.

The ADR approach may be preferable to a traditional "crash course" style of review for a variety of reasons. Time restriction is a fundamental barrier to comprehensive review. Because of the difficulty in keeping up with the expansiveness of information available today, a more efficient and directed approach is needed. Individualized review that starts with the areas of deficit helps the learner narrow the focus and begin customized remediation instead of a blanket A-to-Z approach. Additionally, review that occurs sequentially over time may be preferable to after-the-fact efforts after completion of a program when faculty are no longer available to assist with remediation.

Early identification of content weaknesses may prove advantageous to progressive program success. "Smaller bites" for content achievement and a shortened lapse of time between the introduction of course content and remediation efforts is likely to be more effective in catching the struggling learner before it is too late. Regular feedback keeps learners "on track" and reduce attrition rate by identifying the learner who is "slipping." This approach provides the opportunity to tutor or implement intensified instruction before the learner reaches a point of no return and drops out of the program.

Step I: Proctored Assessment

The ADR program is a method using a prescriptive learning strategy that begins with a proctored, diagnostic assessment of the learner's mastery of nursing content. The topics covered within the ADR program are based on the current NCLEX-RN® Test Plan. Proctored assessments are administered in paper-pencil and online formats. Scores are reported instantly with Internet testing or within 24 hours for paper-pencil testing. Individual performance profiles list areas of deficiencies and guide the learner's review and remediation of the missed topics. This road map serves as a starting point for self-directed study for NCLEX® success. Learners receive a cumulative Report Card showing scores from all assessments taken throughout the program—beginning to end. Like reading a transcript, the learner and educator can monitor the sequential progress, step-by-step, an assessment at a time.

Step II: Modular Reviews

A good test is one that supports teaching and learning. The score report identifies areas of content mastery as well as a means for correction and improvement of weak content areas. Eight review modules contain concise summaries of topics with a clinical overview, therapeutic nursing management, and client teaching. Key concepts are provided to streamline the study process. The ATI modules are not intended to serve as a primary teaching source. Instead, they are designed to summarize the material relevant to the licensure exam and entry-level practice.

Learners are taught to integrate holistic care with a critical thinking approach into the review material to promote clinical application of course content. The learner constructs responses to open-ended questions to stimulate higher-order thinking. The learner may provide rationales for actions in various clinical scenarios and generate explanations of why the solution may be effective in similar clinical situations. These exercises serve as the venue to shift from traditional didactic memorization of facts toward the use of analytical and evaluative reason in a client-related situation. The clinical application scenarios involve the learner actively in the problem-solving process and stimulate an attitude of inquiry.

These exercises are designed to provoke creative problem solving for the individual learner as well as collaborative dialogue for groups of learners in the classroom. Through group discussion, learners discover the technique of elaboration. Learners use group dialogue to increase their understanding of nursing content. In study groups, they may pose questions to their peers or explain various topics in their own words, adding personal experiences with clients and examples from previously acquired knowledge of the topic. Together they learn to reframe problems and assemble evidence to support conclusions. Through the integration of multiple perspectives and the synergy involved in the exchange of ideas, this approach may also facilitate the development of effective working relationships and patterns for lifelong learning. Critical thinking exercises for each topic area situate instruction into a problem-solving environment that can capture learners' attention, increase motivation to learn, and frame the content into an application context. Additionally, the group involvement can model the process for effective team interaction.

Step III: Non-Proctored Assessments

The third step is the use of online assessments that allow users to test from any site with an Internet connection. This online battery identifies specific areas of content weakness for further directed study. The interactive style provides the learner with immediate feedback on all response options. Rationales provide additional information about the correctness of an answer to supplement learners' understanding of the concept. Detailed explanations are provided for each incorrect response to clarify topics that learners often confuse, misunderstand, or fail to remember. Readiness to learn is often peaked when errors are uncovered; thus, immediate feedback is provided when learners are most motivated to find the answer. A Performance Profile summarizes learners' mastery of content. Question descriptors for each missed item are used to stimulate inquiry and further exploration of the topic. The online assessment is intended to extend the learners' preparation for NCLEX® in a way that is personally suited to their deficiencies.

Step IV: ATI-PLAN™ DVD Series

This multi-disk set contains more than 28 hours of nursing review material. The DVD content is designed to complement ATI's Content Mastery Series™ review modules and online assessments. Using the ATI-PLAN™ navigational points, learners can easily find the content areas they want to review.

Recognizing that individuals process information in a variety of ways, ATI developed the ATI-PLAN™ DVD series to offer nursing review in a way that simulates the classroom. However, individuals viewing the ATI-PLAN™ DVDs can navigate through more than 28 hours of material to their topics of choice. Nursing review is available at the convenience of the learner and can be replayed as often as necessary to ensure mastery of content.

The regulation of personal learning goals and the ability to plan and pursue academic intentions are the keys to successful learning. The expert teacher is the one who can determine individual learning needs and appropriate strategies to master learning. The ADR program is an efficient method of helping students prepare for the nursing licensure exam using frequent and systematic content review directed by the identified areas of content weakness. The interactive approach for mastery of nursing content focused in the areas of greatest need is likely to increase student success on the licensure exam.

ATI's ADR method parallels the nursing process in concept and in design. Both provide a framework for solving actual and potential problems purposefully and methodically. Assessment ADR-style is accomplished with ATI's battery of proctored assessments. Diagnosis is facilitated by the individual and group score reports the proctored assessments generate. Planning for improving performance in identified areas of weakness incorporates ATI's modular review system. Implementation begins with modular review and culminates in use of ATI's online assessments to validate improvement. Evaluation is reflected in the score reports, and performance can then be strengthened or further improved with the ATI-PLAN™ DVD series. Just like the nursing process, ATI's ADR prescriptive learning method often leads to specific, measurable results and highly desirable outcomes.

Table of Contents

1 Leadership and Management 1

Leadership Styles Typically Found in Organizations 2
Characteristics of the Effective Leader 3
Levels of Management 3
Characteristics of a Manager 4
Communication Skills and Competencies of a Manager 4
Scope of Practice 4
Effective Management Functions 5
Skills of the Nurse Manager instead of Roles 5
Management by Objectives and by Exception 7

2 Management and Planning Process 10

Phases of Planning 10
Elements of a Plan 11
Barriers to Implementation of a Plan 11
Critical Issues that Arise During Planning 12
Types of Plans 12
Decision-Making Process 13
Case Management 15
Critical or Clinical Pathways 16
Consultation 17
Discharge Planning 17

3 Leading Change 20

Types of Change 21
Stages of Change 21
Strategies for Implementing Change 21
Barriers to Change 22
Characteristics of Effective Change Agents 22
Forces that Motivate Change 23
Forces that Inhibit Change 23
Typical Groups or Responders to Change 23
Interventions for Dealing with Resistance to Change 23
Roles of Nurse Manager 24
Functions of the Nurse Manager 24

4 Management and the Organization 26

Types of Organizational Structure 27
Elements of Organizational Approaches 27
Organizational Process 28
Organizational Culture 28

5 Health Care Delivery Systems 30

Health Care Settings 31
Health Care Providers.. 32
Health Care Professional Competencies 32
Factors Affecting Health Care Delivery 33
For-Profit and Not-for-Profit Delivery Systems 33
Integrated Delivery System 34
The Five "R"s 34
Reimbursement 35
Key Reimbursement Terminology... 37

6 Management and the Team Approach 41

Working with Teams... 42
Types of Delivery Systems 42
Managed Care and the Nurse... 43
Shared Governance 44

7 Resource Management.. 47

Fiscal Planning 48
Types of Budgets... 48
The Budgetary Process... 48
Classification of Costs.. 49
Compensation for Services... 49
Reports and Variances 50
Resource Allocation... 50
Advantages and Disadvantages of Various Staffing Methods 52
Standards of Productivity and Staffing 53

8 Human Resource Management.. 56

Recruitment 57
Management Functions in Indoctrination 60
The Work Environment... 60
Conflict Management 64
Performance Appraisal 66

9 Time Management.. 75

Why Is Time Management Important?.. 75
Diagnosis: What Are Your Time Management Problems? 75
Taking Action 76

10 Delegation 79

Benefits of Delegation 80
Considerations for Selection of Appointee 80
Effective Ways to Delegate 80
Barriers to Effective Delegation 80
Delegation As It Applies to the Health Care Organization 81
Health Care Organization Issues 81
Delegation Process 81
The Five Rights of Delegation 82
Liability and Delegation 83
Tasks That Can Be Delegated by Registered Nurses 83

11 Quality Improvement 85

Aspects of Health Care Quality 86
Continuous Quality Improvement (CQI) 86
Standards and Other Tools 87
Benchmarking 88
Utilization Review 89
Culturally and Linguistically Appropriate Services (CLAS) 89
Accreditation 89
Magnet Status 90
Staff Education 90
Management and the Learning Environment 91
Mentorship for Adult Learning 91

12 Ethical Issues 93

Moral Frameworks (Theories) 94
Moral Principles 94
Values 95
Method for Professional Decision-Making 96
Common Ethical Issues Involving Nurses 96
Ethical Responsibilities of the Manager 96
Nursing Codes of Ethics and Standards of Professional Performance 97
Ethics Committees 97

13 Legal Issues 99

Law Basics 99
Civil Law in Health Care Delivery 100
Regulation of Nursing Practice 107

Critical Thinking Exercise Answer Keys 110

References 135

CHAPTER 1

Leadership and Management

Key Points

- Leadership and management have important effects on health care organizations and the delivery of health care services.
- Leadership styles include autocratic, democratic, laissez-faire, bureaucratic, participative, charismatic, transactional, transformational, connective, and shared. Effective leadership requires vision, influence, and power.
- The three approaches of management are first-level, middle-level, and upper-level.
- Critical management functions include leadership, planning, organizing, directing, controlling, recognition, development, advocacy, coordination, staffing, reporting, and budgeting.
- A supervisor has the authority to hire, transfer, suspend, promote, assign, discipline, and terminate employees.
- Effective nurse managers are outcome-oriented.
- The key components of an organization are structure, process, and outcomes.
- Other important issues are culture, conflict, use of assertiveness, and advocacy.
- Change is a critical process experienced daily in organizations. Barriers to change must be considered during the change process.
- The nurse manager is accountable for excellence in practice, management of resources, compliance with standards, strategic planning, and facilitation of cooperative and collaborative relationships.
- Followership is an integral part of effective leadership.
- Effective managers look for multiple strategies to build cohesive teams in the practice setting.

Overview

Leadership and management roles are commonly believed to be the responsibility and function of professional nurses in positions of authority. It is important to understand that all nurses who are client advocates display qualities and engage in activities of leading and managing in everyday practice situations. Nurses function in this role by planning and providing care to clients; working in collaborative environments with clients, families, and other health care professionals; or contributing to the organization in positions of responsibility.

Leaders influence others to work together to accomplish the goals that are consistent with the mission, values, and purpose of the organization. A predominant characteristic of leaders is the vision and the ability to assertively motivate others to fulfill the group or organization's objective, to inspire confidence, to facilitate change, and to mentor others. Leaders increase productivity by maximizing work effectiveness through inspiration and empowerment of the workforce. They build reciprocal trust relationships with followers and demonstrate competency in change processes. The primary determinant of harmony and satisfaction in the workplace is leadership. Critical thinking skills and good communication are essential elements of effective leadership. Leaders do not just happen; leadership is earned, not gained through appointment, and is a process learned over time and through experience.

Managers are employees to whom the organization has given authority, power, and responsibility for establishing standards, directing the work of others, and evaluating that work. Managers' tasks include implementing organizational policies; controlling resources; setting goals; making decisions; and planning, prioritizing, and solving problems. In a managerial role, the nurse initiates and implements change. The management role is supportive of the leadership function, sharing the vision and affirming the goals of the organization. Good managers must have leadership abilities, and leaders often develop managerial skills. Leadership is the key to effective management.

Leadership Styles Typically Found in Organizations

Autocratic (authoritarian, directive): The leader makes the decisions for the group and assumes people are externally motivated and incapable of independent decision-making. This style of leadership is most effective in emergencies (e.g., a fire on the unit).

Democratic (consultative): The leader encourages group discussion and collaborative decision-making. Individuals are empowered to make decisions to support the leader.

Laissez-faire (nondirective, permissive, ultra-liberal): The leader operates under the premise that the group is internally motivated and needs autonomy and self-regulation. The leader assumes a "hands-off" approach.

Bureaucratic: The leader presumes the group is externally motivated and does not trust self or others to make decisions. Instead, the leader relies on organizational rules and policies, taking an inflexible approach.

Charismatic: The leader's personality evokes strong feelings of commitment. The charismatic leader tends to form an emotional relationship with group members.

Transactional: This leader is focused on the day-to-day tasks necessary to achieve the organizational goals. The leader provides incentives to promote loyalty and performance (e.g., gives a nurse a weekend off in exchange for her working a night shift).

Transformational: The leader fosters creativity, risk-taking, commitment, and collaboration by empowering the group to share in the organization's vision. The leader facilitates individual independence, growth, and change, and converts followers into leaders through shared values, honesty, trust, and continued learning.

Connective: The leader promotes collaboration and teamwork within the organization and among other organizations in the community.

Shared (participatory, inclusive): The leader assumes that a professional work force contains many leaders. No one person is considered to have more knowledge or ability than anyone else. Members of the group are drawn into the decision making. For example, staff nurses and the nurse manager share a vision of their preferred future. The nurse manager develops the vision independently after receiving group input.

Characteristics of the Effective Leader

- Vision is the mental image of a desirable and possible future state. It is the basic ingredient of leadership.
- Influence is an informal strategy used to gain cooperation without exercising formal authority. It is based on a trusting relationship and often involves persuasion and good communication skills.
- Communication skills adaptable to a variety of constituencies are essential to a good leader.
- It is essential for the leader seeking workplace harmony and collaboration to earn the trust of employees. In order to exist, trust must be a reciprocal relationship between the leaders and the employees.
- Power is the ability to influence or to exert actions that result in changes in attitudes or behaviors of followers.

  Reward power is based on incentives offered by the leader.

  Coercive power is based on fear of retribution or withholding of rewards.

  Legitimate power is granted by a specific position or role (e.g., a nurse manager for a critical care unit).

  Expert power comes from the respect others have for the leader's abilities, knowledge, or skills.

  Referent power refers to admiration of and respect for the leader's character or success.

  Charismatic power is the leader's ability to attract and inspire followers.

- Power is an important element of the change process and of leadership and management.

Levels of Management

The manager's job is to accomplish the work of the organization. Roles and functions may vary with the type of organization and the differing levels of management. Titles for these managers vary from one health care organization to another. For example, a health care organization may have a nurse executive or director of nursing, nurse managers, and charge nurses.

First-level managers manage the work of non-managerial staff and the day-to-day activities of a specific work group.

Middle-level managers supervise several first-level managers and serve as liaisons between them and upper-level managers.

Upper-level managers are organizational executives who are responsible for establishing goals and strategic plans for the organization.

Characteristics of a Manager

Nurse managers need to be result- or outcome-oriented. Confronting economic, clinical, and professional issues on a daily basis requires the manager to use problem-solving and team- building methods. Nurse managers interpret and enforce unit and hospital policy procedures and mandates, thus acting in the role as gatekeeper. Self-awareness and evaluation are critical to success. An effective manager will use a combination of leadership styles.

Effective managers encourage "followership" to build successful health care teams. Followership is a healthy, self-confident use of individual behaviors that contribute to positive client care and family outcomes that guide health care team success. Followership is an active process that leads to meeting organizational and clinical outcomes. The nurse, or nurse manager, acquiesce certain tasks such as planning and direction-setting to individuals with the specific skill sets needed to complete the assignments.

Communication Skills and Competencies of a Manager

- Critical thinking
- Communication
- Networking
- Managing resources (e.g., budgeting and staffing)
- Enhancing employee performance (e.g., mentoring)
- Team building
- Evaluating effectiveness and efficiency
- Delegating
- Clinical and organizational expertise
- Flexibility
- Collaboration (interdisciplinary)
- Coordination
- Change agent
- Staff development

Scope of Practice

The nurse manager is accountable for:

- Excellence in the clinical practice of nursing and delivery of care.
- Organization, coordination, and control of staff, fiscal, and other resources.
- Institutional/organizational compliance with standards of care (professional, regulatory, governmental).
- Strategic planning.
- Facilitating cooperative and collaborative relationships with all health care providers to ensure effective client care.

The nurse manager supports and works toward attaining the health care organization's goals and ensuring that employees do the same. The nurse manager, however, needs to participate in the process of goal development using the skills and experience to ensure the provision of effective care and the consideration of the needs of the staff.

Effective Management Functions

Leadership: Providing guidance, direction, and motivation

Planning: Assessing a situation, establishing goals, developing a plan of action

Organizing: Establishment of the formal structure of authority through which work subdivisions are arranged, defined, and coordinated for the defined objective

Communication: An interactive process of information transfer from person to person that is essential in any relationship. Verbal communication is influenced by the speaker's tone, inflection, and volume, while nonverbal messages are expressed through gestures, posture, facial expressions, and eye contact.

Directing: The continuous task of making decisions and implementing those decisions through the work of others

Controlling/Monitoring: Includes evaluating and rewarding others for their work

Recognition: Positive feedback, promotion, salary change

Delegation: Entrusting others with tasks they are competent to perform

Development: Staff education

Advocacy: Representing staff and clients

Coordination: Ensuring that inter-related parts of the work are completed

Staffing: Ensuring that appropriate staff is available to do the work

Reporting: Keeping those to whom you are responsible informed

Budgeting: Ensuring the availability of needed resources (e.g., staff, supplies, and equipment) to meet needs

Problem Solving: Conflict resolution

Critical Thinking: Using high cognitive processes that include decision making, problem solving, creativity, and clinical judgement

Skills of the Nurse Manager

Conflict Management

Conflict cannot be avoided; however, it can be constructive instead of destructive. Conflict serves as a warning signal that some aspect of the inner structure of the group is not functioning effectively, and can point to potential areas for change. Conflict management requires a realistic view of the possible collaborative outcome. The goal is to reach a solution that meets everyone's needs, is agreed upon, and then implemented. This is not always simple or possible to do, thus a give-and-take negotiation is frequently required.

Sources of conflict may include:

- Individual issues and values
- Organizational communication
- Organizational values
- Lack of staff recognition and participation
- Financial instability
- Differences in values among U.S.-educated and foreign-educated nurses
- Cultural biases
- Language differences among nursing staff members

Conflict can increase stress and decrease productivity. Coping with conflict on a long-term basis, particularly if ineffectively dealt with, may lead to physical and psychological problems. Managers may see increased staff absenteeism, morale problems, turnover, and decreased productivity from their employees.

Some of the typical methods of coping with conflict include:

Avoidance/Withdrawing: Failure to acknowledge that a conflict exists; "fight or flight" concept

Compromise: Both sides yield something to the other.

Confrontation: Bringing the problem out in the open is an attempt to resolve it positively.

Collaboration: All parties work together to mutually solve the problem.

Competition: Parties make concerted efforts to achieve their individual desired outcome, no matter what the cost.

Accommodation: Parties work together to solve the problem, but in a nonassertive manner that neglects personal concerns. Ultimately, one party compromises.

Negotiation: A key response in which the parties give and take on the issues.

Assertiveness

Assertive behaviors are essential for effective managerial function. Activities characteristic of the assertive manager include: goal-setting, consistent implementation of action toward the goal, and the ability to evaluate the response and make adjustments as necessary. Key tasks for an assertive style of management include:

- Communicating clearly and consistently
- Knowing yourself
- Taking responsibility
- Proactively managing conflict and confrontation
- Avoiding defensiveness
- Setting reasonable limits
- Recognizing faults and being honest about them but not being overly apologetical
- Dispersing conflict in an emotional situation until rational discussion can occur
- Saying "no" without being aggressive or feeling guilty
- Recognizing that change is good and cannot be avoided

Advocacy

Advocacy is to plead on the behalf of another. Nurse managers are advocates when they act in the best interest of clients and their nursing staff members. Here are some examples of advocacy within a health care setting:

- A nurse educates a client and the family about their legal rights regarding treatment options.
- A nurse manager develops a budget that protects staffing levels or provides funds for educating the staff regarding new treatments and medication.
- A nurse manager goes to the nurse executive to ask for a specific program or change that will benefit clients.

- The nurse executive advocates for the nursing staff members as they participate in activities related to overall management of the health care organization.

Remember that all nurses are expected to act as client advocates. Nurses are responsible for protecting each client's human and legal rights, and ensuring that the client's needs are met. Nurses need to provide a safe environment for clients, and protect clients from injury resulting from possible adverse effects of medications and treatments. It is also the nurse's role to educate clients and their families about their rights, and to assist clients if these rights are threatened or violated.

To be an effective client advocate, the nurse needs to be aware of cultural differences among clients and must respect the cultural beliefs of each client. Also, the nurse must try to provide a professional medical interpreter for a client who does not speak or understand English, or who has limited English proficiency (LEP).

Clients' rights are constantly evolving due to changes in federal regulations and accreditation standards, and nurses must stay informed. Most institutions have established a formal statement addressing clients' rights. These statements include the basic principles of human dignity, integrity, honesty, confidentiality, privacy and informed consent. Fairly recent additions to clients' rights include accessible health care and self-determination through advanced directives. The admissions process in the majority of hospitals includes providing clients with literature informing them of their rights. It is important for nurses to discuss concerns with clients and to answer their questions about their rights.

In addition to protecting the rights of the individual client, nurses need to advocate for the rights of all clients by becoming professionally and politically active. Nurses should speak out against policies or actions that might endanger the well-being of clients as a group.

Supervision

A supervisor is a person who has authority from an employer to hire, transfer, suspend, assign, discipline, and terminate employees. Identification of this authority is particularly important in labor relations. A staff registered nurse (RN) may be "supervising" or monitoring the nursing activities of licensed practical nurses (LPNs) or unlicensed assistive personnel (UAP). However, this is not the same as the definition of a supervisor as the RN simply ensures that tasks are completed effectively and safely. In most cases, this RN would not be in a position to terminate employment of supportive personnel. Employment decisions are within the scope of practice of the nurse manager, other administrative staff, or agency policy.

Management by Objectives and by Exception

- Management by Objectives (MBO) is a managerial method that focuses on identification of objectives and measuring results. The objectives represent expectations. Individuals, small groups, or the entire organization may use MBO. Objectives are identified and written. After they are implemented, the results are evaluated. This evaluation is then used to identify new objectives. MBO is a method that can involve all levels of staff.
- Management by Exception (MBE) is a management approach that focuses on responding only when a problem occurs. This approach tends to focus more on negative feedback, and is generally not an effective managerial method.

Critical Thinking Exercise: Leadership and Management

1. Identify the type of leadership power that is used in the following situations:

   a. M.T. is considered to be the unit's source of any information on diabetes. You go to her to ask for help about a newly admitted client with complicated diabetes.

   b. The nurse manager in labor and delivery is viewed as the "dictator" by her staff and is known throughout the hospital as someone who is very controlling and restrictive.

   c. R.B. was hired for the position of nurse manager for a home health agency.

2. M.S. has just taken a new position. She will supervise all of the medical units (four total). Each unit has a nurse manager. What level of management is M.S.'s new position?

Situation: You are applying for a nurse manager position for a neonatal unit in a large academic medical center.

3. The position description details the scope of practice for the Nurse Manager position. What would you expect to be the scope of practice for the management position and what management functions would you expect to be listed in order for you to accomplish what the nurse manager position entails?

4. What skills and competencies would you want to emphasize during your interview?

5. You know that you will encounter conflict in your new position. How would you cope with conflict? Would you use any of the coping methods mentioned in this module? Knowing how you have managed conflict in the past, decide how you might handle the following situation: The census for your unit has been low, prompting the need for your nurses to float to other units. You overhear some of your nurses complaining about floating and how they are not enjoying work anymore.

6. Explain the concept of followership.

7. The nurse manager will be implementing a new form of electronic charting. Two nurses, the evening charge nurse and a staff RN are highly skilled in the field of computer technology. They have attended classes at the nearby university on topics related to health services and technology. The nurse manager delegates the task of orienting all nursing staff and troubleshooting the new electronic charting procedure to these two RNs. They are given time to complete the task and the part-time nurses will pick up hours of work to facilitate task accomplishment of the RNs' new duties.

   a. Has the nurse manager delegated the task appropriately?

   b. What strategies is the nurse manager employing to facilitate this project?

CHAPTER 2

Management and Planning Process

Key Points

- Planning is the deliberate determination of a course of action to achieve the specified goal(s). The process involves deciding what needs to be done, when, by whom, and why.
- Decision-making requires that you know where you are going, which makes planning critical.
- The major types of planning are strategic, operational, contingency, and project.
- The planning phases are: project selection, development of a solution, implementation of the plan, and monitoring, correcting or changing the plan.
- Critical issues that arise during planning are conflict, advocacy and response to change.
- Elements of a plan are purpose or goals, and objectives such as relevant research, supportive data, budget, timeline, strategies, responsibilities, monitoring and evaluation, and follow-up.
- Quantitative decision-making tools assist the nurse manager and entire team in making important decisions.

Overview

If you do not know where you are going, you will probably end up somewhere else. What does this statement tell you? Planning is critical for successful accomplishment of an objective and fulfillment of a vision. The manager's role is to formulate and implement the plan for achieving the goal of the institution. Planning is the process of realizing the vision. Outcomes-based criteria must be established that will allow you to evaluate the results. Decision-making is integral to the planning process for achieving the intended outcome.

Phases of Planning

Planning is dynamic, in that it has many interactive loops and is not a neat, sequential process. When involved in a project, it is often necessary to go back and forth between the different planning phases. Factors impacting the planning process include:

- Selecting reasonable purpose/goals and criteria/objectives
- Choosing solutions and implementation methods
- Making decisions based on evaluative data

The use of evaluative data is very important and making the careful selection of required data is a significant part of the project. Healthcare organizations tend to be overloaded with data. Do not forget to consider data that is already collected and pertinent to the project. Planning requires that you consider alternatives and think creatively.

The phases involved in the general planning process are:

- Project selection
- Development of a solution plan
- Implementation of the plan
- Monitoring and evaluating/correcting the plan

Implementation of the plan requires cooperative involvement and staff "buy-in." In fact, this element alone can make or break the successful implementation of the project. Other factors that are important during implementation are resources (such as supplies and equipment), financial needs, timelines, individual roles, communication, and the environment.

Elements of a Plan

- Purpose/goals and objectives/criteria
- Supportive data: advantages and disadvantages
- Budget and allocation of resources
- Timeline
- Strategies/interventions
- Identification of responsibilities
- Implementation
- Monitoring and evaluation
- Follow-up

Barriers to Implementation of a Plan

- Poorly defined organizational mission and values
- Lack of understanding or misinformation about the planning and implementation phases
- A focus on daily tasks rather than visionary perspective for future plans
- Competing priorities
- Complexities of implementation strategies
- Distractions and interruptions
- Internal resistance
- Inadequate skills, training, education, ability, or knowledge necessary to implement the task
- Personal disorganization and ineffective time management skills
- Ineffective delegation of duties
- Poor match between appointee and the delegated task
- Inconsistent management style and lack of managerial control
- Lack of role delineation

Critical Issues that Arise During Planning

- Conflict
- Assertiveness
- Advocacy
- Change
- Competition
- Personal motives

Types of Plans

Strategic

Strategic planning focuses on long-range operations and clarifies the organization's beliefs and values. The purpose is to define the future of the organization and develop a plan of action to achieve change. The goal is to improve the organization's effectiveness and efficiency by accurately implementing the visionary activities. Each component of the organization develops plans, which are compiled to form the basis of the strategic plan. Development of the strategic plan requires that the organization has a sense of direction, understands its strengths and weaknesses, and has the creativity to maximize its strengths.

- Elements of a strategic plan are:
  - Mission/vision, purpose/goals, and objectives
  - Appraisal of organization's strengths and weaknesses
  - Needs analysis
  - Application for subsidiary funding or grant awards
  - Marketing plan
  - Budget and cost analysis
  - Activities to promote the program and communicate the benefits
  - Satisfaction surveys
  - Interviews with clients
  - Qualitative or quantitative research
- Phases of strategic plan:
  - Strategic plans are reviewed annually by the key leaders in the organization and should include input from other staff. The plan may need to be revised as goal attainment is evaluated throughout the year. The strategic planning process is proactive, vision-directed, outcome-based, and oriented toward growth and change. Phases of the strategic planning process generally span 3-5 years and include:
    - Development of a mission statement and declaration of philosophy, purpose/goals, objectives, values, and purpose
    - Determination of the need and impact of the deserved action or change
    - Identification and analysis of critical organizational issues (e.g., strengths and weaknesses, environmental issues, competition and threats, opportunities, financial status, relationships with the community)

- Identification of strategies for action to attain goals
- Implementation of specific plans for action
- Evaluation of progress or satisfaction of purpose/goal; adjusting the approach as necessary

Operational

An operational plan focuses on the day-to-day operation of the organization. Emphasis is placed on what factors are needed to get the job done. As different components within each organization develop plans of their own, organizations will end up with many operational plans. These plans must be flexible and evaluated regularly. They should not conflict with the overall strategic plan, but rather serve as the building blocks for the strategic plan, supporting the organization in meeting its mission and goals.

Contingency

A contingency plan is developed for specific problems that may occur, so that the organization can be proactive. Examples of hospital-based contingency plans include what the hospital will do when it must close its emergency room due to the census (e.g., no hospital beds available); how to respond to a natural or internal disaster; and how to handle a nursing shortage.

Project

Project development should be seen as an opportunity for growth, not a burden. Some staff members may view a project as something that they are told to do and do not want to do. When a project is first considered, there are factors that will affect the content and result. These factors include internal and external policies; state and national regulations; professional issues and standards; accreditation; organization (structure, process, and culture); financial issues, resources, and the organization's mission and goals.

The first question you might ask is, "What is a project?" It is some action or series of actions that is needed to solve a problem, institute a change, and create/develop a product or program. Some examples of projects are developing a new procedure for processing admissions to the psychiatric unit; instituting a women's health program; changing the documentation for critical care clients; developing a case management program for a health care agency; and developing a client education program for postpartum mothers who only stay in the hospital for 24 hours.

Decision-Making Process

Factors Affecting the Process

Many factors affect decision making; however, the most common are:
- Availability of resources (financial, staff, supplies, equipment)
- Mandate for a change
- Authentic need for a decision or change
- Leadership and management style
- Involvement of staff
- Past history with change

Phases of the Decision-Making Process

Decision-making is an essential component of the manager's daily role. A successful decision maker: 1) thinks creatively to develop new ways to solve problems; 2) is willing to take risks; and 3) is sensitive to other people and situations. Successful decision-making requires critical- thinking skills that include both intuitive and analytical approaches. An organized, structured approach is the best way to make quality decisions because it reduces trial and error. The traditional problem-solving model is probably the most widely known, but it is time consuming and lacks an initial goal-setting step. Table 1 compares the steps of the traditional and managerial problem-solving process with the nursing process. The comparison shows how closely these processes parallel one another. It should be noted that goal setting or identification of objectives is not always clearly evident. The key to quality decisions is not which process is used, but how the process is used. Setting goals, writing clear objectives, and using logical thinking are critical components in any decision-making process.

Table 1: Decision-Making Process for Nurse Managers

Traditional Problem-Solving Process	Nursing Process	Managerial Decision-Making Process
Identify the problem	Assess	Set objectives
Gather data to analyze causes and consequences	Problem identification Nursing diagnosis	
Explore alternative solutions	Plan	Search for alternatives
Evaluate alternatives		Evaluate alternatives
Select the appropriate solution		Choose
Implement the solution	Implement	Implement
Evaluate the results	Evaluate	Follow-up

Decision-Making Tools

To assist managers in the decision-making process, there are a number of tools that provide order and direction in gathering and processing information. It should be noted that these tools or models do not guarantee the final decision. They act only as guides in the decision-making process. Each has limitations and may not be appropriate for all situations.

Decision tree: A decision tree is a graphic tool that helps organize the key elements of the situation. All of the relevant data is plotted on the tree and each alternative strategy is plotted as a branch on the tree. Sub-branches are identified and labeled as risk factors and other critical factors to consider.

Decision grid: A decision grid or matrix helps the decision maker to compare and contrast each of the alternative solutions. For example, across the top of the grid, factors such as financial impact, time element, risk factors, and required resources might be listed. Along the vertical axis of the grid, the different alternatives are listed. In this manner, the different alternatives are easily compared. The decision grid might be useful, for example, in deciding which type of nursing care model would be most effective for a specific unit.

Numerical scoring: Each identified strategy is assigned a numerical value based on criteria such as probability of success, cost, time, etc. A decision is based on the highest score. This approach is relatively simple and allows the decision maker(s) to analyze all the alternatives concurrently.

Program evaluation and review technique (PERT): The PERT flow diagram is a popular tool for determining the time element in the decision-making process. Estimating project completion in a timeline format is useful for planning a complex activity. For example, finish times ranging from the most optimistic to the most pessimistic are estimated for developing and implementing a new treatment program. The flow chart shows critical tasks that must be completed before the project can continue.

Payoff table: This tool is used for decisions that can be made solely on the basis of fiscal impact. For instance, a nurse executive might approve the following request for continuing education (CE) if the education department director could show they would either make a profit or break even (achieve a budgetary break-even point). Here is the possible scenario:

> The education department wants to offer a CE session on how to use new intravenous (IV) pumps. They would need to buy supplies ($150 for IV tubing, IV fluids, etc.), pay for an expert speaker (a $1,000 honorarium), and use two of their personnel to coordinate the event ($350, at $25/hour for 7 hours each). Their total costs would therefore be $1,500. They would market the session to surrounding hospitals, long-term care facilities, and schools of nursing. The charge per participant would be $50.

> To achieve a budgetary break-even point, 30 people would have to register for the session (30 x $50 = $1,500).

> If <30 people registered, a loss would be incurred.

> If >30 people registered, a profit would be made.

Case Management

The case management concept is not new to health care. However, case management is more frequently used today as a strategy to control the rising cost of health care. This method of delivering client care is based on outcomes and specified cost management strategies. Case management incorporates a multidisciplinary approach to providing and documenting care. The purpose of case management is to:

- Better coordinate care, particularly for clients with complex health care needs
- Improve the efficiency of care and resources needed to provide care
- Improve the quality of care delivered

The primary function of case managers include:

- Communicating and negotiating with other health care professionals, clients and family members
- Coordinating care
- Coaching
- Advocacy

This collaborative process uses case mangers to determine that the appropriate services and resources are rendered at the appropriate time. The case manager may be a nurse, social worker or other health care professional. The care manager is not a direct care provider, but instead assesses and implements guidelines to assist in cost containment. Examples of settings where a case management approach may be implemented include:

- Extended hospitalization for the premature infant with complex medical needs
- Provision of home oxygen therapy for the client with chronic emphysema requiring home health oxygen therapy
- Provision of care for the client with AIDS who requires complex medical care and costly medication
- Provision of care for the client with schizophrenia who requires ongoing mental health services and medication in order to maintain function in the outpatient setting
- Provision of care to clients with multiple conditions

If a case manager is not involved in the care of a client and the client requires multiple resources, the nurse can initiate a case conference that includes care providers from all disciplines. During the case conference, care providers outline the client's major care requirements. The processes of assessment, diagnosis, planning, implementation and evaluation are similar to those used in case management. By initiating a care conference, the nurse is acting as a client advocate to ensure that all of the client's needs are appropriately and adequately addressed.

Critical or Clinical Pathways

A clinical or critical pathway is a standardized, multidisciplinary plan that maps out the expected course and time frame of treatment for clients with similar problems or diagnoses. The nurse and other team members use these critical pathways to monitor an individual client's progress around the clock. Thus, caregivers use one clinical pathway as a monitoring and documenting tool to help them track the clinical course for clients. The clinical course for clients is based on the average and expected lengths of stay in a health care facility. Important aspects of the critical pathway include discharge planning, client education, consultations, activities, nutrition, administration of medicines, diagnostic tests and treatment.

Because clients are individuals with their own specific problems, some clients will deviate from the critical pathway plan. Such variances in client outcomes may be either positive or negative, depending on how the client responds to treatment. A positive variance occurs when a client progresses more rapidly than expected. A negative variance occurs when the activities on the clinical pathway are not completed as predicted, or the client does not meet the expected outcomes. Variances can result from one-time causes, from changes in the client's health, or from other health complications unrelated to the primary reason the client needs care. The nurse's responsibility is to correct the variance — or to justify the actions taken to manage the critical pathway deviation.

Critical pathways benefit nurses and clients in many ways. Better communication results in increased continuity of care. Novice health care providers have a structure to follow. Clients are involved in the planning process. Critical pathways are excellent teaching tools. The entire health care team is involved in all phases of client care. Discharge planning and teaching are initiated early in the client's stay. Health care institutions also use critical pathways to evaluate the cost of care for different groups of clients.

Consultation

Consultants are specialists who have the expertise to identify various ways to solve a problem. Consultants are also used when the exact problem remains unclear. A consultant can assess and identify the problem objectively and outline a method for resolution.

Nursing consultation is sought when nurses have identified problems they cannot solve using their own knowledge, skills and resources. Consultation increases the individual nurse's knowledge of the problem and helps the nurse acquire skills and obtain resources to help solve the problem. After the consultation, the nurse may be able to resolve similar problems in the future.

The first step in the consultation process is to identify the general problem area. Second, the nurse should contact an expert who can help solve the problem. Third, the nurse provides the consultant with pertinent information and resources about the problem area. This includes a brief summary of the problem, methods used to resolve the problem so far, and the outcome of those methods. Other resources include the client's medical record, nurses and other members of the health care team, and the client's family. Fourth, the nurse discusses the consultant's findings and recommendations with the consultant. Finally, the nurse incorporates the consultant's recommendations into the care plan, and then implements the plan.

Discharge Planning

It is essential to start discharge planning early in the client's hospitalization. Discharge planning involves:

- Assessment of the quality of the person's support system (e.g., which family members or friends are involved in the client's care)
- Evaluation of the person's ability to learn and perform self-care activities
- Assessment of the person's psychophysiologic condition

Teaching prior to discharge is very important. Provide the client with clear written guidelines on self-care procedures, lifestyle changes, diet, medication administration, exercise, required environmental modifications, possible complications and follow-up care.

Some clients maly need health care assistance once they go home. If necessary, refer the client and family to community agencies and resources for home care.

Critical Thinking Exercise: Management and Planning Process

1. You are working on a committee for your home health agency. The purpose of the committee is to develop a plan for meeting client needs during major catastrophes or inclement weather. What type of plan are you developing?

2. The hospital has noticed on client satisfaction surveys that clients do not feel that their pain is being adequately addressed and attended to during their hospital stay. As the quality improvement nurse, you have been asked to implement "pain" as the fifth vital sign on the client's chart. As you develop this project, consider each of the four phases of planning and state what you might do during each of the four phases.

3. A committee at the home health agency begins to work on a plan for inclement weather. What must be included in the plan? Identify the elements of the plan and some specific information related to each element applicable to this committee's purpose.

4. The nurses on the Oncology Unit are planning a health fair in the community for Lung Cancer Awareness Day. The budget for their portion of the fair is $3,000. They will provide Registered Nurses to take health histories, arrange for primary care provider presentations on the subject, and disseminate educational pamphlets to attendees. The general public will be charged $5 per person. How many paying participants will be needed to break even?

5. You are a nurse on the Medical-Oncology unit and frequently encounter ethical dilemmas associated with end-of-life issues. What quantitative tool for objective decision-making will assist you in making difficult decisions involving ethical dilemmas? Why?

6. What is the purpose of using case management?

CHAPTER 3

Leading Change

Key Points

- A clear definition of mission, values, purpose, goals, and objectives is essential for leading and effecting change.
- Leaders develop vision and set goals for change within organizations, groups, and among individuals.
- Managers implement the vision of the leader through activities such as planning, organizing, budgeting, controlling, and problem solving.
- Many people naturally resist change because it represents upheaval, disruption, uncertainty, and instability. The nurse leading change may anticipate this common attitude and facilitate an understanding of the benefits for change.
- In order for change to be accepted, it should be based on an actual need or problem; however, not all change results from a need or a problem.
- Driving forces that motivate change are based on the belief that change will improve a situation, impart benefit, and impact gain.
- Restraining forces that inhibit change stem from perceptions of loss, negative past experience, misunderstanding of the benefit of change, and exaggerated focus on the barriers to implementation of an operational plan.
- Strategies to implement change depend on the individual or group attitudinal and behavioral responses. Internal and external forces promulgate the need into action.
- Communication is the key to successful implementation of change.
- Team synergy effects change more than the action of an individual's efforts.
- To produce change, the nurse leader engages in active listening, compassion, cooperation, and a commitment to problem resolution and goal attainment.
- Stages of change:
  - Perception of the need for change and discontentment for status quo
  - Formulation of a strategy for implementing change
  - Integration of the plan while supporting the team
  - Evaluation of plan effectiveness and necessary adaptations
- Strategies to promote change:
  - Empirical-rational
  - Power-coercive
  - Normative-re-educative

Overview

Change is a complex process of altering, revising, or causing deviation from an established pattern. Change is a primary function of nurses in virtually all health care delivery settings. The nurse in the role of change agent initiates, motivates, and implements improvement. The challenge for nursing today is to identify changes to benefit clients, health care organizations, and the nursing profession. An insightful and proactive approach is necessary to cause improvement in the care delivered to clients, as well as our practice environment. The effective change agent possesses the expert authority, skills, knowledge, and power to facilitate needed change.

Types of Change

Unplanned change occurs without any control or effort by a person or a group.

Planned change is an intended, purposeful attempt or proactive plan by an individual ("change agent") or group to influence its own status quo or that of another system or person.

Covert change occurs without the individual's awareness.

Overt change occurs with the person's awareness.

Developmental change occurs as a result of the physical and psychosocial changes that occur during the life cycle or course of time.

Stages of Change

Kurt Lewin (1951) contributed significantly to our understanding of the change process. He identified three phases that the change agent must initiate before a planned change can occur.

Unfreezing is the first phase of the change process in which the change agent creates discontent with the current situation. In other words, during this phase, the change agent elicits feelings of concern or anxiety regarding the status quo and creates an increased awareness of the need for change. This process also involves a thorough assessment of the group's general interest in change and the degree of motivation of the group members.

Movement is the second phase of planned change and involves identification of strategies and alternatives for change. The change agent also identifies strategies that ensure the driving forces for change exceed the restraining forces. Identifying and overcoming resistance may be a long process and this component of the movement phase may take a great deal of time in order for all members of the group to assimilate the change.

Refreezing is the final phase where the change agent continues to support individuals as they continue to adapt and integrate the new system.

Strategies for Implementing Change

There are three commonly used strategies for implementing change. The appropriate strategy for any situation depends on the power of the change agent and the amount of resistance expected from the group members.

Empirical-rational strategy assumes people are rational and are receptive to change when adequate facts are provided. This method focuses on reason and knowledge and is often used for technological changes. For example, if someone explained to you that you could save $20 every month by using a different light bulb, then you would be more inclined to change because it would save money.

Power-coercive strategy assumes that change occurs as a result of an individual's desire to please a supervisor, or out of fear of losing one's job, or receiving some other type of punishment. Using our example of the light bulb, the husband decides to change to the different light bulb because his wife has refused to pay the light bill unless he makes the switch.

Normative-reeducative strategy assumes that change will only occur after attitudes, values, and relationships are altered. This approach involves the members of the group in planning for change. For example, the entire family has a series of discussions about the family budget and examines how much money is spent on electricity. Because they value family time, they decide to approach the problem with a new attitude on cost containment — planning to apply the money they save on electricity to the summer vacation account.

Barriers to Change

Emotional reactions: Fears, biases, and emotive responses due to a lack of understanding

Perceptual issues: A lack of perceived need, resulting in resistance to change

Economic threat: Fears of termination of job, salary cut, lack of a promotion, or loss of benefits

Social threat: Fears about changing the social structure or relational patterns of the work environment

Characteristics of Effective Change Agents

- Excellent communication and interpersonal skills
- Project expertise
- Knowledge of available resources
- Problem-solving skills
- Teaching skills
- Respected by those involved
- Self-confident, risk takers
- Inspire trust in themselves and others
- Able to make decisions
- Broad knowledge base
- Good sense of timing
- Ability to be flexible
- A good sense of humor
- Ability to motivate others to participate
- Ability to acknowledge an individual nurse's enthusiasm concerning a change, while helping that nurse allow other nurses to react to a change at their own speed

Forces that Motivate Change

"Driving Forces"

- Belief that the change will bring economic gain
- Belief that the change will improve the situation
- Perception of the change as a challenge
- Visualization of the future impact that the change will have
- Potential for growth, recognition, achievement, and/or improved relationships

Forces that Inhibit Change

"Restraining Forces"

- Need for intellectual and emotional security (low tolerance for change)
- Lack of time or energy
- Fear that something of value will be lost (e.g., threat to job security)
- Misunderstanding of the meaning and implications of the change
- Failure to see the "big picture"
- Perception that the change will not have any benefits ("will not work")
- Perceived loss of freedom to engage in desired behaviors/activities
- Past experiences with change that had a negative effect

Three strategies for dealing with driving and restraining forces:

- Increasing the number or strength of the driving forces
- Decreasing the strength of the restraining forces
- Combining the first two strategies

Typical Groups or Responders to Change

Innovators: Thrive on change

Early adapters: Respected by peers; sought out for advice and information about changes

Early majority: Prefer what was done in the past, but will accept new ideas

Late majority: Openly negative; agrees to change only after others have accepted

Laggards: Openly express resistance; prefer keeping traditions

Rejecters: Actively oppose and may sabotage change to interfere with the change process

Interventions for Dealing with Resistance to Change

- Educate staff regarding the need, benefit, and process for change.
- Communicate with resisters to find out their reasons for opposing the change.
- Facilitate staff members "buying into" the change, and adopting it as their own.
- Clarify and correct inaccurate information.
- Present the negative consequences of resistant behavior (e.g., poor client care).

- Emphasize the positive consequences of the behavior change in terms of how the person or group will benefit.
- Be open to suggestions/revisions, but be clear about what must be maintained.
- Foster a climate of trust and support.
- Encourage interaction between supporters and resisters. Encourage supporters to empathize with resisters and relieve unnecessary fears.
- Seek advice from expert consultants (preferably external) to help employees work through sudden or particularly difficult changes in the workplace.

Roles of Nurse Manager

Planned change is a deliberate effort to make something happen. Planning, coordinating, and implementing change requires well-developed leadership and management skills. Leadership roles and management functions in planned change include:

- Recognition of the need for planned change
- Establishment of goals, objectives, and purpose for change
- Identification of alternatives and resources to implement change
- Demonstration of risk-taking behavior
- Flexibility in planning and goal setting
- Anticipation of resistance to change
- Implementation of creative problem-solving strategies
- Modeling a positive attitude toward challenge and opportunities for growth
- Demonstrating creativity in problem solving
- Seeking input from group members
- Fostering an environment of trust and security
- Providing adequate feedback and information throughout the change process
- Objective communication and relational skills
- Using appropriate change strategies to modify behavior of group members, as needed
- Functioning as a respected authority figure and change agent

Functions of the Nurse Manager

Human Resources: Staffing, performance appraisals, professional licensure, certification, or other documentation for competency-based practice

Fiscal Resources: Budgetary allocations, unit expenses, and product control

Informatics: Client classification systems and client data

Health Care Environment: Adherence to Occupational Safety and Health Administration (OSHA) and Joint Commission on Accreditation of Healthcare Organizations (JCAHO) requirements; environment characterized by professionalism

Critical Thinking Exercise: Leading Change

1. Staffing on a busy medical-surgical unit has been inadequate to address client acuity levels. Nursing administration is implementing 12-hour shifts instead of 8-hour shifts to cover busy parts of the workday. Using each of these approaches, how would the unit manager's approach in the change process differ?

    a.   Power-coercive strategy

    b.   Empirical-rational strategy

    c.   Normative-re-educative strategy

2. The nursing unit where you work is changing to a different intravenous infusion pump.

    a.   Identify some specific activities that should occur during the "unfreezing" phase of this change.

    b.   Discuss what needs to happen to enable change as you examine the possible driving and restraining forces.

3. You are responsible for implementing a change in documentation on your unit by introducing a new system for documentation of nursing activities. You know that many staff members have complained that this will just add more work, and it is just another example of making a useless change. The staff has felt overworked all year and its members see it as more work. Would you describe the staff responses as a "driving" or "restraining" force for change? What might you do to increase success with the change?

CHAPTER 4

Management and the Organization

Key Points

- An organization is a group of people working together to achieve a shared goal.
- Organizational structure describes the design for working relationships, methods of communication, decision-making process, and designation of responsibilities within the organization.
- The mission of an organization is the stated purpose in the community.
- The philosophy of an organization is the expression of beliefs and values that are fundamental to its operation.
- A vision statement is the iteration of the future orientation and direction of an organization, including a summation of the mission, values, and philosophy.
- Objectives are statements of behavioral activities for achieving the desired outcome of the organization.
- Organizational function is the way that interactions usually occur within an organization.
- The approach to delegation of authority within an organization may be centralized, decentralized, matrix, hybrid, or self-governance.
- An organizational chart is a schematic representation of the structure of the organization, including positions, departments, functions, and reporting relationships. It defines the lines of authority, responsibility, and accountability for goal attainment.
- Chain of command identifies the path of authority and accountability within an organization.
- Span of control refers to the breadth of responsibility and authority for directing the action of others within the organization.
- Organizational culture refers to the prevailing attitudes, feelings, relational patterns, communication, and interactions that influence the operations within an organization.

Overview

An organization is a group of people with roles and responsibilities to serve a common purpose and achieve a shared goal. The mission, philosophy, values, and goals, as well as structure and people within it, influence the nature of the organization. Dimensions of the social system within an organization include the individuals, environment, and structure; the behavior of people within this system is affected by the complex interaction of these dimensions. Bureaucracy is a primary characteristic of an organization, particularly denoting the formal aspects of the organization.

Types of Organizational Structure

To view the structure of an organization, it is best to organize a chart of its departments, positions, functions, and the relationship they have with one another. The framework for delineating the authority, responsibility, decision-making and accountability is defined in the organizational structure. A traditional structure uses vertical relationships or the chain of command (who reports to whom). Today, many organizations use a structure that emphasizes horizontal relationships rather than the traditional vertical structure.

Bureaucratic: A formal, centralized hierarchy characterized by clear rules and regulations, and labor subdivided into specialties.

Matrix: A formal vertical and horizontal chain of command characterized by fewer rules and levels of hierarchy where expertise is centralized at the customer level.

Flat: A formal, decentralized chain of command without the hierarchy; decisions are made in the work area.

- Shared governance: A flat structure with accountability, responsibility and authority given to the nurse delivering the care.

Hybrid: A mixture of the formal structures

Elements of Organizational Approaches

Various types of organizational approaches are used in health care today. The approach used provides structure for where within an organization decisions are made. A centralized approach focuses tasks and authority in one location or source. Decisions are made at the top and flow down. Decentralization spreads tasks and authority throughout multiple components within the organization. Decisions are made at or close to the client-care level. Examples of each may be found in how staff education is organized in a hospital. For example:

- A centralized organizational approach gives a staff development department the responsibility for staff orientation and education throughout the hospital.
- A decentralized approach gives this responsibility to the units. The division of responsibility gives nurse managers more independence in the management of their units.
- A matrix approach represents a type of centralized structure that designates dual authorities that are responsible for product and function-related tasks. The focus of a product manager in the health care setting is outcome-based client care. The functional manager handles the provision of care and actions required to produce the outcome or product.
- A hybrid approach describes the structure that operates with the characteristics of different types of structure.
- Self-governance is a type of organizational structure that involves the participatory management of managers and staff members. The delineation of responsibility, decision- making, and accountability are shared. This design is often successful for enactment of a professional practice model.

Each organization has a formal or official aspect, as well as an informal aspect. It is important to understand the function of both. As you review an organizational chart that describes the formal positions and hierarchy, it is helpful to know the informal structure as well. This informal structure identifies which staff members are leaders, even if they do not hold a formal title in the hierarchy, or which of the managers is more powerful than the others for reasons other than authority. Power within the informal structure is often based on expertise, knowledge, skills, or relational characteristics.

Organizational Process

An organizational process focuses on how the organization functions. Particularly important to its infrastructure are the operations of communication, decision-making, policies and procedures, job performance, goal attainment and results, quality improvement, budget, and future plans. Nurses participate in all aspects of the organizational process, from the staff level to the upper levels of the organization. The organization's mission/vision statement, philosophy, goals, and objectives are an integral part of the organizational process.

Mission Statement: Clarifies the organization's unique purpose

Vision Statement: Clarifies the future direction the organization will take

Philosophy: Describes the organization's beliefs and values

Goals and Objectives: Indicate how the organization plans to attain its mission and philosophy

Organizational Culture

An organizational culture is reflected in the way the collective members of a select group think, behave, and share expressed meanings, norms, and values. The organization's rituals become extremely important to the group. When a person becomes a member of a particular culture, certain aspects of thinking, behaving, and communicating are shared and then become the mode of behavior by that person while in the organization.

Factors Influencing Organizational Culture
- Structure and process
- Communication, both formal and informal (e.g., use of memos, e-mail, gossip, accessibility of information, private conversations and secrets are kept from the larger groups, time needed for staff to know about changes, effective communication, information overload)
- Acceptance of new members/staff
- Willingness to allow new members to offer suggestions or new ideas
- Management's willingness to include staff in the change process
- Morale
- Staff turnovers
- Feedback

The organization's mission statement and goals reveal what the organization thinks about itself and its staff; however, it is important to match what is written with what is demonstrated. The goal is to have a consonant culture, one that emphasizes the sum of its parts, rather than its many separate parts or dissonant culture.

Critical Thinking Exercise: Management and the Organization

1. You have decided to accept a new position as charge nurse on a pediatric unit at a small rural hospital. Discuss the type of control you will have based on the organizational chart below.

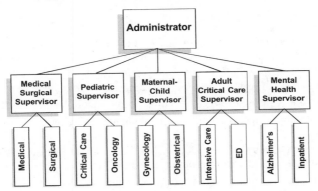

2 Think of some questions you might ask to assess the organizational culture of the institution that you are considering as a place of employment.

3. As the nurse manager you are responsible for ordering supplies for the unit such as paper, pens, etc., as well as client supplies. You have decided to delegate this responsibility to one of the unit secretaries. The secretary has decided to enlist the help of the morning charge nurse when ordering client supplies since the unit secretary is not completely familiar with client needs. Would you consider this process of delegation and spread of authority an example of a decentralized or centralized organization?

4. Compare and contrast organizational structure and process.

CHAPTER 5

Health Care Delivery Systems

Key Points

- Health care delivery systems are organized to deliver health care services with three purposes: provide health promotion and illness prevention, diagnosis and treatment, and rehabilitation and health restoration.
- The three levels of services are primary care, secondary care, and tertiary care.
- There are many different types of acute and non-acute health care settings.
- There are many different health care providers who are members of the health care team.
- With a complex health care system many factors affect its results (e.g., access, managed care, increase in number of uninsured, etc.).
- Not-for-profit health care organizations are more recently restructuring to for-profit organizations.
- The five "R"s in health care organizations are re-engineering, redesigning, regulating, right-sizing, and restructuring.
- Cost containment and reimbursement issues have had major effects on health care delivery.
- Health care systems have moved from a retrospective payment system to more of a prospective system.
- The major payment sources are the government (Medicare and Medicaid) and third- party payers (includes managed care organizations).
- Managed care organizations focus on economic control, gatekeeping, and primary care.
- Capitation is a prepayment to a provider and is a critical method used in managed care.
- Working with teams provides an opportunity for staff to work together collaboratively.
- Nursing care delivery systems have changed over the years. Some examples are: primary care, team nursing, and the functional case method.
- All nurses work in a managed care environment.

Overview

A health care system consists of all the agencies and professionals that are organized to provide health services. Its purposes are to provide (1) health promotion and illness prevention, (2) diagnosis and treatment of illness and injury, and (3) rehabilitation and health restoration. Health care services can be organized according to their complexity:

Primary Care: Health promotion and education, preventive care, early detection, and environmental protection

Secondary Care: Diagnosis and treatment, acute care, and emergency care

Tertiary Care: Long-term care, rehabilitation, and care of the dying

Some health care systems provide all of these levels of care (e.g., large academic medical center that includes acute care, emergency services, clinics, home care, and hospice), while others focus on just one level (e.g., nursing home, wellness clinic for newborns).

Health Care Settings

Health care settings vary in the type of services they offer, their size, location (urban or rural), type of people they serve, and the reimbursement for these services.

Public health: Federal, state, or local government agencies are funded primarily by taxes and administered by elected or appointed officials. Local health departments develop and carry out programs to meet the health needs of groups within the community and the community as a whole. For example, the Centers for Disease Control and Prevention (CDC) provides epidemiological investigations.

Primary care providers' offices

Ambulatory care centers: Offer health care services provided on an outpatient basis (e.g., one-day surgery centers, diagnostic centers).

Clinics: May be inside or outside a hospital and provide a variety of services or specialized services, such as infant immunizations. Some functions of the clinic overlap with primary care providers' offices and ambulatory care centers.

Industrial clinics: Provide occupational health services at work site.

Hospitals: Deliver acute care health services.

Extended-care facilities: Includes skilled nursing (intermediate care) and extended-care (long-term care) facilities. These types of facilities may be inside or outside a hospital.

Subacute facilities: Deliver extensive care to clients just discharged from hospitals but who are still acutely ill, have complex medical needs, or who may require high-tech equipment.

Retirement and assisted-living centers

Rehabilitation centers

Home health agencies

Hospice services

Psychiatric hospitals and community mental health centers

Substance abuse treatment centers

Health Care Providers

Health care providers are also referred to as health professionals, health care givers, or the health care team. These are people from different disciplines who work together to promote client wellness and/or restore health. The following are some examples of health care professionals:

- Professional nurses/registered nurses (RNs), including advanced practice nurses, clinical nurse specialists, and nurse midwives
- Licensed vocational/practical nurses (LVNs/LPNs)
- Unlicensed assistive personnel (UAP), patient care assistants (PCAs), nursing assistants (NAs)
- Primary care providers (PCPs), medical doctors (MDs), doctors of osteopathic medicine (DOs), nurse practitioners (NPs), and physician assistants (PAs)
- Mid-level providers: names that may be given to NPs and PAs
- Primary care provider's assistants (PCPAs): Diagnose and treat certain diseases and injuries under the direction of a primary care provider (in states where PAs are not recognized as PCPs)
- Dentists
- Pharmacists
- Dietitians and nutritionists
- Physical therapists
- Respiratory therapists
- Occupational therapists
- Laboratory and radiology staff
- Social workers
- Case managers
- Spiritual support persons (e.g., chaplains)
- Alternative care providers (e.g., chiropractors, acupuncturists)
- Students

Health Care Professional Competencies

Nurses practicing in the national initiative to improve the health of Americans, as described in the *Healthy People 2010* objectives, provide care that is focused on health promotion and disease prevention. The broad goals (as described by the Department of Health and Human Services) are aimed at increasing the healthy life span for Americans and reducing the disparity of health conditions and services among Americans.

The professional competencies of the nurse are necessary to effect change for improving health care, including:

- Exhibiting ethical behavior in all professional activities
- Assuming a responsibility for fair and ethical practices and personal values
- Ensuring relationship-centered care with respect to the individual and family
- Advocating for client rights
- Communicating effectively with members of the interdisciplinary team
- Contributing to quality-improvement activities and evidence-based practice

- Providing culturally competent care to all members of our diverse population
- Delivering clinically competent care
- Maintaining an emphasis on preventative health measures
- Demonstrating critical thinking skills for creative and effective problem solving
- Incorporating population-based care into practice

Factors Affecting Health Care Delivery

- Problems with access to health care: Eligibility for government programs/ benefits, transportation, hours of operation, number and type of providers
- Introduction and development of managed care
- Increase in the number of uninsured, a growing problem in the U.S.
- Changes in demographics: single-parent families, immigrant populations, lack of extended family nearby
- Increase in the number of older adults with complex health care needs
- Improved technologic advances: computers, organ transplants, genetic engineering, diagnostic procedures
- Increase in the cost of health care: medical care costs have increased more than 400% since 1965.
- Uneven distribution of services: remote and rural areas may not have enough health care professionals to provide needed services
- Increased specialization: contributes to fragmentation of care and increased cost of care; a client may receive care from up to 30 people during a hospital stay.
- Increase in homeless populations: adults and children
- Increased availability of drugs

For-Profit and Not-for-Profit Delivery Systems

- For-profit health care organizations, also referred to as proprietary organizations, have shareholders and sell stocks. The organization is then responsible to the shareholders who expect to make a profit on their investment.
- Proprietary organizations have the same type of reimbursement available as the not-for- profit delivery systems, called voluntary or public health care organizations.

Charitable institutions, government, and churches, as well as the typical reimbursement sources, are considered not-for-profit health care organizations. In the past, there was an expectation that these hospitals served the community and would provide care regardless of the ability to pay. This is no longer true; indigent persons receive health care from Medicaid providers contracted for services.

It is important to recognize that not-for-profit health care organizations must still make a profit to survive, but this profit is not disbursed to shareholders, but rather is re-invested into the health care organization to expand services and maintain the organization.

Integrated Delivery System

Integrated delivery system (IDS) is an approach to health care delivery that is growing. The characteristics of IDS are:

- A focus on providing care across the continuum of care with a network of services.
- The goal of ensuring that those in the system remain healthy.
- Care is provided at the lowest cost.
- Primary care is central to the care provided.
- Care is provided in a variety of geographic locations.

Vertically integrated health care systems offer a spectrum of health care services along the continuum of care—wellness, prevention, acute and chronic care, disease management and rehabilitation, ambulatory care, long-term and home care, and hospice care.

The Five "R"s

Re-engineering the health care organization: Rethinking the organization and changing its processes to improve its performance. Re-engineering produces radical changes for the organization, not a few minor ones. Currently, there are tremendous demands on health care organizations to increase efficiency and improve cost effectiveness of resources and health care delivery. The managed care approach was designed for controlling costs.

Redesigning the work force: Changing how work is done and who does it is a phenomenon sweeping through health care organizations. Traditional roles and activities are being adapted to meet client needs. Important elements when redesigning the work force include staff education, staff involvement, staff skill set, communication, support and reward, and evaluation.

Re-regulating professional practice: Many of the changes that are taking place in health care delivery require a review and revision of professional practice regulation, licensure, and practice acts. Organizations that engage in practices such as telemedicine must address issues related to licensure, scope of practice, and reciprocity. State boards of nursing granting mutual recognition for professional practice handle interstate reciprocity issues. However, to accommodate these provisions, changes in licensure regulations may be necessary. Other modifications to the Nurse Practice Act and state regulatory stipulations are enacted for the prescriptive authority of advanced practice nurses. Even something like being a flight nurse may become difficult when flying over state lines to pick up a client. Nurses who work in more than one state may need to be licensed in those states. If so, the nurse needs to be familiar with the practice act of each state in which they are licensed.

Right-sizing the work force (sometimes referred to as downsizing): Can be a threatening process for staff. Right-sizing determines the number of staff members required to perform a task or fulfill a role/function safely, productively, and competently. The process is difficult to forecast as many of the key variables, such as census, acuity, and resource availability may be uncertain. Inaccurate projection can compromise the quality of care delivered and the integrity of the health care system. Right-sizing also applies to the business of nursing education, e.g., the match of nursing graduates to meet employment demands.

Restructuring nursing education: Changing nursing education has never been easy, but it is critical that nursing education keep pace with the needs of health care delivery systems. Nursing education has two major components: the undergraduate and graduate component, and continuing education for nurses who are in practice and not actively seeking advanced degrees.

Reimbursement

Cost Containment

With increasing health care costs, health care organizations must regularly analyze their costs if they expect to survive as an organization. No one has the magic answer to the complexities of cost containment, but everyone agrees it must be done. In the early history of nursing in the United States, there was little interest or understanding of health care costs. Health care administrators did not seek nurses' advice in developing cost containment strategies or any other aspect of financing health care. Gradual changes in administrative policy necessitated the involvement of nurse executives and nurse managers to reduce generational, dispensary, and operational costs throughout the budgetary process. Deliberate and proactive strategies are needed to educate the nursing staff about the impact of nursing decisions on budget and costs.

Examples of cost containment methods:

- Decrease overtime expense.
- Decrease sick time expenses.
- Use supplies appropriately.
- Prevent equipment malfunction to avoid major repair costs.
- Decrease inventory of supplies.
- Maintain careful account of client care supplies.
- Maintain productivity standards.
- Prevent employee accidents.
- Use acuity systems to determine staffing levels.
- Schedule part-time staff that does not receive benefits as appropriate to unit function.
- Use of unlicensed assistive personnel for non-nursing tasks.
- Redesign nursing delivery system.
- Increased use of computerized documentation.

Prospective Payment

With the reorganization of Medicare/Medicaid programs, the federal government initiated the prospective payment system. This method establishes reimbursement prior to the provision of services through a system using Diagnostic Related Groups (DRGs), which are codes assigned to client diagnoses, procedural care, and extent of services. Health care decisions, particularly institutional and professional providers, length of services, method of and extent of care, and indications for services are determined by third-party payers who maintain decision-making control through payment in advance of service provided. The resultant effect for health care providers (primary care providers in particular) is a compromised control of their own practice situations. Third-party payers "up the ante" to increase compliance to DRG code and designated-care provider lists. Health care providers and consumers publicly express concerns and discontentment with the restrictions and regulations of the prospective management systems.

Payment Sources

Government

Medicare: A federal government health insurance program established under Title XVIII of the Social Security Act for people age 65 and older, and for individuals of any age entitled to monthly disability benefits. Medicare also provides benefits for those with chronic renal disease who require hemodialysis or kidney transplant. It consists of three separate but coordinated programs: hospital insurance (Part A), the costs of physicians and other providers (Part B), and Medicare Plus Choice (Part C), which expands the availability of managed care arrangements for Medicare participants.

Diagnosis-related groups: In efforts to contain medical expenses at the hospital level, Medicare established a disbursement system that administers a predetermined payment for clients with a specific diagnosis (e.g., regardless of the length of stay or cost of services, a hospital would receive a set amount—say $1500—for a client with an asthma exacerbation). Conceptually, clients whose actual expenses exceed the reimbursed amount are counterbalanced by those clients whose actual expenses are below it.

Medicaid: A governmental health insurance program that provides assistance to members of families through the Aid to Families with Dependent Children program and to certain indigent and disabled individuals. The federal government sets broad guidelines for the program, giving states considerable latitude to establish eligibility criteria and to determine what services will be covered. Although coverage varies widely from state to state, each state must provide the benefits identified by the federal government for basic levels of care.

Increasingly, the government contracts with managed care organizations to provide Medicare and Medicaid services to participants. However, many managed care organizations (MCOs) have found that the cost of health care services often exceeds government reimbursement to the provider. As a result, it is not unusual for an MCO to terminate participation in the Medicare or Medicaid program. This has caused problems for participants who have chosen to use a particular MCO covered by Medicare or Medicaid. When MCOs terminate participation in Medicare or Medicaid, participants typically will be required to change health care providers. This is often a frustrating and confusing experience.

Third-Party Payer

Indemnity insurance is the traditional approach to insurance coverage and includes both commercial and self-insurance. Individuals are considered self-insured when they purchase coverage directly, rather than through an employer. In the U.S., about 80% of private health insurance is provided through employers who determine the type of coverage offered to employees. Institutions, agencies, and providers usually contract with MCOs to administer health care services to recipients.

- MCOs focus on the following key elements:
  - Economic control by regulating services provided (by amount and type)
  - Emphasis on preventive care
  - Focus on client populations: (i.e., the members of the plan or managed care organization)
  - Recognition of efficiency
  - Shifting financial risk to the provider: (i.e., The provider is reimbursed a specific amount; if other care is provided for a longer period of time than what has been approved by the MCO, the provider may not be reimbursed.)

There are many different MCO models. Two of the common models are:

Health Maintenance Organization (HMO): An organized system that offers health services to a group of people who are voluntarily enrolled in the program. HMO care is designed to provide care for health promotion and disease prevention. This integrated delivery system offers health care services for participants at a fixed, prepaid premium. The four basic models for HMO services include: group model, network model, individual practice association, and staff model.

Preferred Provider Organization (PPO): Program in which contracts are established with providers of medical care, referred to as preferred providers. Incentives are offered to participants for selecting preferred providers, including lower co-payment and a higher percentage of coverage for services rendered. Services from non-preferred care providers are allowed but at a higher expense to the participant. PPOs are becoming increasingly popular because of greater flexibility they offer to the participant, particularly in terms of selection of providers and hospital facilities.

Point of Service (POS): Program that attempts to combine the freedom of a PPO with the lower cost of an HMO. POSs are similar to HMOs in that people who enroll in a POS are required to choose a primary care provider from within the health care network. However, they are not limited to only those doctors in their network. They can be referred to doctors outside their network by their primary care provider. There is a deductible for out-of-network care and even when that deductible is met, they may still pay a higher percentage of cost and possibly, the difference between what the health care provider charges and what the plan deems "reasonable and necessary."

Key Reimbursement Terminology

Capitation: A prepayment by the managed care organization or insurer to a provider to provide services to enrollees/members of a health plan. This usually is a monthly payment to a primary care provider in an HMO network. The provider may keep the payment even if no care is provided, although no additional payment is received if the client requires more complex care.

Primary Care Provider (PCP): Provider who is responsible for routine health promotion, maintenance, and illness prevention. The PCP is involved with detection of health abnormalities and treatment of common disorders, and referring clients to specialists for more complex care.

Utilization Review: Review of medical necessity, efficiency, and appropriateness of treatment by the third-party payer. Treatment (including medications) may or may not be approved for reimbursement by the third-party payer.

Benefits: The services that are included in a health care plan. Services may be reimbursed if approved by the plan's utilization review.

Premium: Prices or rates that must be paid for insurance coverage. If coverage is an employer plan, the employer typically pays a portion of the premium.

Co-payment: The fixed amount the enrollee/member must pay per office visit, procedure, hospitalization, or prescription.

Deductible: The amount of the health care costs that the enrollee/member must pay per year before the insurer will begin reimbursement (e.g., The first $1000 must be paid by the enrollee/member, then the insurer provides disbursement at a contracted discount for fees exceeding the deductible amount).

Critical Thinking Exercise: Health Care Delivery Systems

1. Identify the factors affecting health care delivery in your community and the effects they may have. Be specific in identifying factors and effects.

2. How have changes in not-for-profit health care affected the delivery of health care in the U.S.?

3. What is the significance of redesigning the work force and why is it important to consider right-sizing when redesigning is done?

4. You have recently become nurse manager for a medical unit. You have been told one of the goals of the unit is to decrease the operating budget. What cost-containment methods might you use?

5. What is the major difference between retrospective and prospective reimbursement, and how might each affect the hospital's or clinic's budget?

6. What is a potential problem that can occur under managed care? Consider the key elements of managed care organizations.

7. You work in a clinic, and you are orienting a new nurse to ambulatory care. How would you describe the role of the primary care provider to the new nurse?

8. Select a unit that you have worked on, either as an employee or as a student. Describe the nursing care delivery system used on the unit.

9. Are the critical competencies required for a nurse who works for an MCO or for a health care organization affected by managed care any different than the competencies required for all nurses? Support your answer.

CHAPTER 6

Management and the Team Approach

Key Points

Types of delivery systems in the health care setting:

- Functional care model
- Team nursing approach
- Modular nursing approach
- Primary nursing concept
- Total client/case management

Shared governance is a health care delivery model that empowers the nurse to perform in a role based on autonomy for professional practice. The nurse functions as client advocate by participating in decision-making activities directly related to the delivery of nursing care. Participatory management involves collaboration with health care team members in peer review and clinical promotion systems.

Strategies for team building:

- Establishing trust
- Performing whatever tasks are required to accomplish project goals
- Supporting and encouraging the accomplishment and contributions of the team and individuals within it
- Communicating openly and consistently (oral, electronic, and print forms)
- Establishing a team identity and feeling of community
- Listening to input of members and valuing their ideas
- Involving team members in the problem-solving process
- Fostering mentorship for professional growth of members
- Clearly delegating roles and duties
- Treating members impartially (bias can be destructive to morale)
- Identifying external and internal sources of negativism and divisiveness affecting the group
- Including members of the multidisciplinary team for decision-making and critical thinking

Overview

In today's health care environment, a critical nursing competency is the ability to effectively work with a group of individuals. The health care team works together toward mutual goals to restore health and promote wellness. This is accomplished through a variety of health care delivery systems including managed care, and alternative nursing care delivery systems such as primary or team nursing. Although different in scope and function, each of these models requires the collaboration of a multidisciplinary team to develop and implement health care. Ideally, this takes place in an environment that supports shared governance where nurses participate in all aspects of the decision-making process.

Working with Teams

A team is a group of interdependent persons working together to accomplish an identified goal or task. For the team to work effectively and efficiently, a spirit of cooperation, collaboration, and clear, consistent communication is essential. Appropriate delegation, feedback, recognition, mutual respect and support, decision-making and problem-solving activities are other key components of the team process. Productivity reflects the effectiveness of the team to meet its goals and objective. Team cohesiveness and individual satisfaction with the role as a team member highly impacts the generativity of the group. The leadership and management style of the nurse manager and administrators is critical in fostering the relationships, roles, and functions of the team to accomplish the mission and values of the organization.

Types of Delivery Systems

Nursing care delivery systems are always changing. Factors that affect these changes are economics, staffing shortages or excesses, philosophies and goals, tasks that need to be accomplished, and the availability of ancillary staff to assist the nurse. Some systems have come and gone. For example, primary care nursing was popular in many areas of the country, but currently has declined in use, largely due to increased costs and growing shortages. The total client care or case method approach is rarely used on most units, but may be used in critical care settings. Why is this so? Many of the tasks needed to support these forms of care can be done in a more cost-effective manner with the contribution of health team members. Typically, a hospital will use a combination of systems.

Examples of Nursing Care Delivery Systems:

Functional care is a task-oriented approach, focusing on jobs to be done. The nurse in charge assigns the tasks (e.g., one nurse may administer medications for all clients on a unit; an aide may take vital signs for all clients).

Team nursing is led by an RN. A team of two or three people provides total care for a group of clients during an 8-hour or 12-hour shift.

Modular nursing is a form of team nursing. Typically these nursing units have fewer clients, smaller teams of nurses, and only licensed nurses practicing on the unit.

Primary nursing is a method of client care delivery where one nurse is responsible for total care of clients throughout hospitalization. Associates provide care on some shifts with the primary nurse coordinating the client's care.

Total client care/case method requires that one nurse be responsible for all of the care for one client during a shift. Though not a common practice anymore, this case method is currently utilized by student nurses as well as critical care units and recovery rooms.

Managed Care and the Nurse

Nurses work in the managed care environment whether they work for a managed care organization or for any other type of health care organization that receives reimbursement. The **critical competencies** for nursing in this environment are:

- Critical thinking
- Collaboration and multidisciplinary relationships
- Communication
- Coordination
- Negotiation
- Leadership
- Delegation
- Evaluation
- Entrepreneurship
- Conflict management

Leadership functions in the managed care environment include:

- Focusing on opportunities rather than threats
- Engaging in innovative and creative change
- Taking risks
- Empowering staff
- Focusing on successes

The nurse may participate in **many roles within the managed care environment**. Some of these are:

- Client advocate
- Client educator
- Provider liaison: Communicates and coordinates with various providers
- Benefits interpreter: Assists clients and providers in understanding reimbursement benefits
- Triage coordinator: Ensures that clients receive the right care at the right time from the right provider
- Quality improvement
- Utilization/resource management: Controls costs by monitoring what care is provided, its purpose, timeliness, to whom, and by whom
- Risk management: Limits the organization's financial risk or loss
- Disease management: Management of the care and cost for a specific disease, such as diabetes or arthritis
- Population-based care: Improves care for a population that has common health needs

- Outcome-based management
- Discharge planning
- Case manager
- Primary care provider: advanced practice nurse, nurse-midwife, clinical nurse specialist

Shared Governance

Shared governance is a professional practice model that empowers the nurse to function in a role involving autonomy, decision-making for client care delivery, accountability, and self- determination. Instead of administrators in hierarchical positions of authority, it is the nurses providing direct client care who make participatory practice decisions. Control for professional practice is functionally based, focusing on quality of care, delivery methods, client advocacy, education, and interactive planning with the multidisciplinary team. Shared-governance models implement peer review and clinical promotion systems for advanced participation in the management of the practice environment in the form of the "clinical ladder." A nursing council or self-governing body provides the overall leadership structure with bylaws for nursing staff. Thus, shared governance supports nurses and administrators in working toward common goals.

Critical Thinking Exercise: Management and the Team Approach

1. Study the nursing care delivery structure below.

    a.   Discuss which type of delivery system it represents.

    b.   What is the role of the individual at the top of the structure?

    c.   What kind of leadership does this method of delivering nursing care suggest?

    d.   Discuss the issues of responsibility and accountability as they relate to this method of care delivery.

    e.   List several advantages and disadvantages of this system.

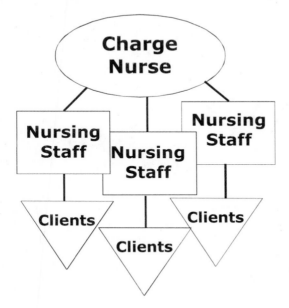

2. You have just been hired as the unit manager for a long-term care facility where the morale of the nursing staff is very low and peer support is virtually nonexistent. Using your knowledge of group dynamics, think of some specific activities that could be initiated to facilitate group participation and teamwork.

3. The Chief Nursing Officer (CNO) in the hospital where you work has supported the team nursing model of client care delivery, but abruptly changed to the functional model of care delivery.

   a. What is the most likely reason for the CNO to abruptly change the client care delivery system?

   b. What are some of the root causes of crises?

CHAPTER 7

Resource Management

Key Points

- A budget is a detailed fiscal plan for carrying out the mission, values, and goals of the organization over a determined period of time.
- The major types of budgets are capital, operating, and personnel.
- The budgetary process is an ongoing one, and it is critical that nurse input is included in the budget.
- The four major phases of the budgetary process are planning, development, implementation and monitoring, and evaluation.
- Costs are classified as fixed, variable, direct, and indirect.
- Compensation methods for services include fee-for-service, per diem rates, case rates, Diagnostic Related Groups (DRGs), capitation, and resources-based relative value scale.
- A variance analysis is the major control process for budget results. Various reports are also used in data analysis.
- Productivity is the ratio of output to input.
- Effectiveness and efficiency are important aspects of productivity.
- Staffing and scheduling are functions of the nurse manager that play an important role in productivity and staff morale.
- Client acuity and census are used in client classification systems to determine staffing needs.
- Scheduling within the health care organization is an ongoing activity of assigning nurse providers to a specified time and location.
- Staffing involves the use of qualified human resources in budgeted positions for delivery of care.

Overview

Resources, such as personnel, supplies, and equipment, are critical to accomplishing the goals and objectives in a health care delivery organization. The two major functions that are important are budgeting and resource allocation (particularly staff). Nursing managers are involved in all aspects of resource management. Successful resource management is supportive of a fiscally strong organization and quality care.

Fiscal Planning

Fiscal planning is the formal plan for managing the financial resources. The balance of expenditures and revenues are projected during a specific period of time, usually annually. Allocation of projected expenses is also part of the budget. Goals and objectives are critical to the development of a realistic budget, as well as the monitoring of budgetary expenses through control procedures.

Budgetary planning is important for:

- Analyzing activities for appropriateness
- Focusing on the future rather than just the present
- Anticipating problems or opportunities in time to deal with them
- Reinforcing motivation to work toward organizational goals

Budget functions are to plan, manage ongoing activities, and control spending. The organization must consider the following questions during all phases of budget planning:

- Do the benefits justify the costs?
- Is the budget consistent with the organization's goals and objectives?
- Is the budget reasonable and realistic?
- Will the organization's revenues be able to support the budget?

Types of Budgets

Capital expenditure: Long-range budgets (usually three to five years) that involve physical changes (e.g., space renovation) and the purchase of major capital items (e.g., major equipment, inventories, and furniture). Priorities need to be established for these items. Assets will depreciate over time.

Operating: Short-term budgets (per fiscal year or annually) that allocate funds for day-to-day activities of the organization. Expenses/costs that are included are utilities, small equipment, medical and non-medical supplies, mortgage/interest/loans/insurance, building maintenance and maintenance of equipment, and personnel expenses. Cost centers are used to track these types of expenses. Projected revenues are also identified in the operating budget. Revenues come from payment sources (insurance/MCOs, government/Medicare/Medicaid, private pay); contributions; and other income, such as interest, rent, and the sale of property or equipment.

Cash: Budget that accounts for the monthly expenditures and receipts to the department and/or organization. Cash flow is an important element. Operations are based on a complexity of fiscal considerations.

Personnel: Budget that allocates expenses related to personnel. Types of expenses are salary, social security, vacation and holidays, education, unemployment, workman's compensation, 401K contributions, and other benefits. The critical aspect of personnel budget planning is forecasting the number of staff needed to provide care for a specified time period (e.g., 24 hours a day, 365 days for hospitals; the forecasting/time period varies for home care and in other types of settings).

The Budgetary Process

The budgetary process is an ongoing one. It begins with the identification of who is responsible for developing and monitoring the budget. Ultimately, the organization's governing board is responsible, but many of the administrative staff members participate and have responsibilities, including the chief executive officer, the chief fiscal officer, nurse executive, and managers. Operational goals and objectives are set that correspond with the organization's mission, goals and objectives, as well as the organization's strategic and operational plans. It is easy to view the budget as another paper report or plan, but it must be a living document, one that changes as needed, and it must be continually monitored. A cost center is a unit or department within an organization that has specified expenses. Examples of this would be the cardiac care unit, the pharmacy department, nursing services, or admissions. Each one would have a budget that would then be used to develop the overall budget for the organization.

There are four major phases in the process.

Planning: Gathering information related to goals and objectives, setting priorities, conducting an environmental assessment, and identifying financial objectives

Development of the budget: Collecting and analyzing data from past budgets, allocating amounts based on priority, and approving the operational and capital budgets

Implementation and monitoring: Analyzing variances and adjustments during the fiscal period, negotiating and revising the budget as necessary, allocating departmental and cash budgets

Evaluation: Obtaining performance reports and analyzing efficiency

Classification of Costs

Fixed: A cost that does not change with volume, which is typically the number of clients. Examples of fixed costs are installment payments for equipment and overhead expenses.

Variable: A cost that changes based on volume. Examples of variable costs are those items used in the operating room, which would change based on the type and number of cases, medications, and, in some cases, staff costs.

Direct: Costs that can be identified for a specific service (such as the cost of the physician's time to perform the service) or product (such as laboratory tests or medication).

Indirect: Costs that cannot be linked or associated with any specific service or product. Office supplies are a good example. For example, it is difficult to say that the use of office supplies is associated with the revenues or income associated with treating 10 cardiac clients.

Compensation for Services

Fee-for-service: The provider charges for services given and is paid by the insurer (or in some cases, the client may pay, but that is less common). This method was the traditional payment method, but is not used as much today.

Per diem rates: Payment that is fixed and based on each day of service, such as $600 per day in the hospital.

Case rates: Payment that is based on the type of case, such as a flat fee for an appendectomy or vaginal delivery.

Diagnostic Related Groups (DRGs): Classification system implemented by the federal Medicare system. DRG categories are used to assign predetermined reimbursement based on the client's medical diagnosis, age, complications, procedures, and other factors.

Capitation: Prepayment per enrollee/member of the plan/MCO to a provider who will then provide specific services, when required, to the enrollee/member. This is usually a monthly payment. If the enrollee/member does not require any services, the provider still keeps the payment. The incentive is to provide less care, rather than more care. This payment method is very common with managed care organizations.

Resource-Based Relative Value Scale (RBRVS): Method used by Medicare, in addition to DRGs. It is used to determine payment for primary care provider services both for procedures and cognitive services (e.g., office visits).

Reports and Variances

Various types of analysis reports that are important in the budgetary process for health care organizations include:

Budget variance report: Describes the status of the budget, what has been spent, and the revenues. A monthly review of the budget is critical in order for an organization to stay on target with the budget. Is the unit spending too much money or below what is expected? These are the variances, the difference between the projected and the actual expenditures in the budget. Managers need to analyze them and determine the causes for the variances. Adjustments may need to be made in the budget, or in the implementation of the budget. Are revenues below what was expected? For example, are there fewer admissions? This can be a major problem for management.

Productivity report: Provides data about the number of staff hours worked per units of service (such as client days or client visits) in terms of allocation of human resources.

Payroll report: Cites employee earnings and hours worked per pay period and considers factors such as vacation and sick time.

Supply variance report: Lists the utilization of supplies and compares it with the budgeted amount.

Resource Allocation

Productivity

Productivity is the ratio of output (products and services) to input (resources consumed). It is important to maximize productivity of resources to preserve the quality of products and services. Factors affecting input are the characteristics of the staff (e.g., experience, stability, interpersonal communication, time management, variable or fixed staffing), and client factors (e.g., age, acuity level). Other factors include the extent of the treatment setting, unit layout, equipment, supplies, and management. Factors that affect output are acuity, client satisfaction, medical records, and client education. Examples of output are the number of emergency room visits, primary care provider office or clinic visits, deliveries, in client admissions, meals served to clients, home visits, and days spent in the hospital. Assessment of productivity requires reviews of the budget, client acuity system, personnel and levels of staffing, client satisfaction, and quality improvement monitoring.

For greater cost effectiveness, some health care facilities that are located in the same community use horizontal integration strategies to provide services to clients. For example, one facility may provide food services to another facility in the community, while the facility receiving food services provides laundry services in exchange.

Effectiveness and efficiency are important elements of productivity. Effectiveness is taking the necessary steps to achieve objectives. It is a managerial goal. Critical sources of data about effectiveness include quality improvement data, performance appraisal, evaluation of nursing care provided, and data from external reviews, such as the Joint Commission on Accreditation of Health Care Organizations. Efficiency is doing the right things correctly. It integrates effectiveness and economy, in other words, meeting the outcomes with the minimum resources to reach the goal.

Staffing and Scheduling

Staffing and scheduling are important functions that directly impact the quality of client care. Staff members are concerned about their schedules, workload, and the amount of time and staff that are available for the clients. Scheduling is done in many different ways. Scheduling may be centralized, done by a nursing service or a specific office for the entire health care organization; or decentralized, which means the divisions or units of the organization do it. A third type of scheduling is self-scheduling, whereby staffing criteria are developed and mutually agreed upon by the staff. Staff members create the schedule themselves, which often requires negotiation and cooperation of the persons involved. Self-scheduling has been very successful in many settings due to the autonomy and self-determination involved. Additionally, self-scheduling facilitates work attendance.

Factors Influencing Staffing Needs

Considerations for staffing are based on a complex array of factors, including volume of services required; complexity and intensity of care; availability; skill level; and qualification of providers. Staff mix is the skill level and ratio of individuals providing professional services for client care. Due to the nursing shortage in recent years, the mix is changing to include the increased involvement of unlicensed assistive personnel (UAPs) and client care assistants (PCAs). This model is often referred to as team nursing, since a team of nurses with varying levels of education and responsibility take care of a group of clients. For example, in a team model, the RN may be responsible for the care of 15 clients with the help of unlicensed assistive personnel, whereas in primary care nursing, the same RN may have a client load of only six. The census, which is the number of clients admitted for services, is an important consideration for staffing a unit. Cost-containment strategies that limit the provision of services in the hospital setting has led to increased acuity in the secondary and tertiary care settings. Demands on staff are directly related to the severity of illness; complexity of services needed to meet the needs of the client; volume of services; and extent of psychosocial support and education. Client classification systems, which determine client needs based on defined criteria, are used to allocate staff to provide the care. For example, to increase productivity when staffing is limited, staff may take orthostatic blood pressure readings only for those clients who are at risk for hypertension.

Staffing Methods

Fixed staffing: Determined by a specified, projected maximum workload requirement. An example is the typical hourly schedule for an 8-hour or 12-hour shift.

Full-time equivalent (FTE): Represents the services required for the equivalent of 2,080 hours annually or 36 to 40 hours per week.

Flex-time: Represents the variations in scheduled hours from the traditional 8-hour shift. For example, four 10-hour shifts per week; three 12-hour shifts per work week; or the Baylor plan, that staffs for weekends, or two 12-hour nights, and considers the position full time. Other flex-time modified Baylor plans have included working five 12-hour shifts in a row and then having nine days off, or working seven 10-hour shifts in a row and having seven days off. In each case, the nurse is considered full time and gets full benefits.

Specialization: Grouping clients according to medical needs, such as neonatal intensive care, critical care, orthopedic, renal dialysis, etc. Expert staff is assigned to care for these groups of clients with special needs.

Alternating/rotating shifts: Working more than one type of shift (e.g., scheduled days and evenings within a single work period).

Block/cyclic: The same schedule is repeated over and over. For example, an individual might be scheduled to work six successive days followed by two days off. The schedule repeats itself every six weeks.

Variable (including on call): Use of client needs to identify the mix and number of staff required. This requires some type of client classification system. Staff levels will fluctuate based on client needs. The organization may use part-time and outside agencies to assist with increased staffing needs. This method focuses on identifying the peak workload time periods to ensure that needs are met during those times. Examples of clinical specialties where this is more common due to fluctuating workload/census are labor and delivery and emergency rooms.

Advantages and Disadvantages of Various Staffing Methods

There are many variations in staffing patterns, each with distinct advantages and disadvantages. Staffing policies of the individual institution primarily determine staffing schedules.

Scheduling Method	Advantages	Disadvantages
Permanent	Fewer health problems, less absenteeism, greater job satisfaction, can plan social life	Day shift most desired, evening and night shifts staffed mostly with new graduates
Flex-time	Improves weekend coverage and reduces turnover, more time to relax on consecutive days off	12-hour shifts correlated with greater fatigue
Alternating/ Rotating	This type of scheduling could be advantageous if entire work group or teams that are compatible are rotated	Increased stress and physical complaints, reduced work quality, higher turnover, rotation of personnel is disruptive to work groups
Block/ Cyclic	Reduces fatigue, sick time reduced, schedule is known in advance, staff treated fairly, decreases floating, improves continuity of care	Somewhat rigid schedule
Variable	Census determines staffing, less need to call in unscheduled staff	Dependent on a valid, reliable client-classification system

Standards of Productivity and Staffing

Staffing requirements are based on a standard unit of measure for productivity. One of the most commonly adopted standards in many hospitals is a client classification system. This method of quantitatively estimating client care needs and staffing requirements to provide necessary care is based on census and acuity level. Once an appropriate system is developed and adopted by the institution, the number of nurse care hours can be assigned for each classification. The standard formula for calculating nursing care hours (NCH) per patient day (PPD) is the number of nursing care hours worked in 24 hours divided by the client census.

$$\frac{NCH}{PPD} = \frac{\text{Nursing hours worked in 24 hours}}{\text{Client Census}}$$

For example, the client census is 20; the number of nursing care hours needed for each acuity level and the number of clients at each level is as follows:

Category l = 2.3 hours (7 clients)

Category ll = 3.0 hours (4 clients)

Category III = 4.2 hours (4 clients)

Category IV = 5.1 hours (4 clients)

Now we can calculate the number of nursing care hours per client: The total number of nursing care hours equals 65.3 hours. This was determined by multiplying each category (acuity level) by the number of clients falling into that category (Step 1), and adding all of the hours from the four categories together (Step 2). Then, the total number of nursing care hours is divided by the number of clients (Step 3).

Step 1

Multiply each category (acurity level) by the number of clients falling into that category.

Do the math:

Category I   = 2.3 hrs. x 7 clients = 16.1 hrs.

Category II   = 3.0 hrs. x 4 clients = 12 hrs.

Category III = 4.2 hrs. x 4 clients = 16.8 hrs.

Category IV = 5.1 hrs. x 4 clients = 20.4 hrs.

Step 2

Then add all of the hours from the four categories together.

16.1 + 12 + 16.8 + 20.4 = 65.3 hours

Step 3

Divide the total number of nursing care hours (65.3) by the number of clients receiving care (20). This equals 3.26 hours per client for that day.

$$\frac{65.3 \text{ (Nursing Care Hours)}}{20 \text{ (Client census)}} = 3.26$$

Nursing units are generally budgeted for so many hours per client per day. Calculating the number of nursing care hours required for any given day can assist the manager in determining if the unit is understaffed or overstaffed.

Critical Thinking Exercise: Resource Management

1. Why is it essential to consider goals and objectives when developing a unit budget?

2. Explain the nurse manager's role during each phase of the budgetary process.

3. Compare fee-for-service compensation with capitation.

4. As a director of nursing, you are reviewing your home health agency's budget reports. What reports would you review and why?

5. What is the difference between effectiveness and efficiency?

6. As you consider productivity for a hospital unit, what are three examples of outputs that would be important to review?

7. If you have (a) some staff members who work 8-hour shifts based on a five-day workweek, (b) some who work evenings and nights in the same pay period, and (c) others who work the 12- hour shifts based on a three-day workweek, what types of scheduling do these staff members have?

CHAPTER 8

Human Resource Management

Key Points

- Human resource management involves tasks like interviewing, hiring, coaching, retention of staff, and performance evaluation/appraisal.
- It is essential to hire individuals from diverse cultures who will be able to serve the client population.
- A position description is an outline of the qualifications and expectations for a job.
- There are many motivation theories (e.g., Maslow's hierarchy of needs, Alderfer's modified need hierarchy, Argyris's psychological energy, McClelland's basic needs, Herzberg's motivation-hygiene, McGregor's theory of X and Y, and Skinner's positive reinforcement theories).
- Job satisfaction is important in recruitment and retention of staff, productivity, quality of care, and morale. The work environment is important for job satisfaction.
- Mentoring is an important component for career development, especially for women, and has become more prevalent in the past 20 years.
- Burnout occurs when a person is no longer effective in his/her job due to stress, boredom, role strain, or job dissatisfaction.
- Absenteeism may result from a variety of causes: unplanned events, poor morale, low personal motivation, role stress, job dissatisfaction, family demands, illness, jury duty, or other unanticipated factors.
- Staff education is critical today with the ever-changing health care needs and treatment methods.
- Turnover is costly for the health care organization.
- Many health care organizations have unions.

Overview

The primary functions of human resource management (once referred to as the "personnel department") involve interviewing, hiring, coaching, retention of staff, and performance evaluation. In some organizations, staff education falls under the auspices of human resource management. Staff education may be included as part of a specific department, such as nursing service or client care. Many elements affect the selection and retention of staff, including motivation, job satisfaction, the work environment, burnout, competency, discipline, staff education, and unionization.

Recruitment

Position Description

A position description is a formal definition of the qualifications, duties and responsibilities of an employee written in the standardized format adopted by the institution. When developing the job description, the nurse's professional competencies are influenced by nurse practice acts, state regulations, professional and institutional standards, and codes of ethics. Job descriptions should be reviewed annually and any time the nature of the job changes.

During the recruitment and selection process, position descriptions aid in determining the fit between the candidate and job expectations. They serve to communicate to team members the roles, duties and functions for the shared goal of the group. Additionally, clear descriptions not only enhance the efficiency of the job at hand but also aid in delegation of responsibilities to team members. Position descriptions are used as a measure for performance appraisals by specifying criteria for evaluation.

Steps in the Recruitment Process

Recruitment of qualified staff members is critical to the success of the health care organization. It is important to hire staff members at all levels (nurses, physicians and administrators) who are bicultural and bilingual. A diverse staff that represents the local population will be able to provide care to clients from different cultures and ethnic groups. Listed below are steps the nurse manager takes to find the right people for the right job.

- The interviewing process begins by defining and describing the position and performance expectations. Clarity in identifying the competencies, roles, and job-related functions in the preliminary phase of hiring a prospective employee is a key element for retention after recruitment.

- Advertisement, which takes place either outside the institution or by internal posting, by word of mouth (the most effective method), or through informal invitation, occurs prior to the interview.

- The nurse manager or person in the human resource department reviews the application, resume or curriculum vitae, and letters of reference as determination of the applicant's qualifications, education, and experience relevant to the position.

- Establishing rapport is enhanced by creating a comfortable environment and non- threatening dialogue with the applicant. Human resources, a panel of interviewers, or the nurse manager, depending on the size and structure of the organization and the nature of the position, may handle the initial screening.

- During the selection process, an important step is posing interview questions to determine whether the applicant's values, skills, and experience are commensurate with the mission, goals, and objectives of the institution. Direct and specific questions regarding the candidate's ability to think on his/her feet in a situation likely in the job may help guide the interviewer to selection.

- Responding to the applicant's questions is integral to the mutual fit between candidate and employer. Typically, the discussion includes information regarding the position and role expectations, organizational structure and chain of command, salary and benefits, scheduling, and unique aspects or demands of the position. The interviewer should always have a copy of the position description available during the interview.

- The interviewer creates closure by thanking the applicant for his/her time, for interest in the position and organization, and by informing the person what follow up is needed after the interview.

Effectiveness of Interview Process

A primary limitation of the interview is its subjectivity. Although the interview is often viewed as reliable because of its interactive nature, in reality it is full of bias. Interview tools are evaluated on two measures: 1) reliability and 2) validity. If an interview or assessment tool is said to be reliable, it measures the same thing consistently each time it is used. Even though the tool may be reliable, it may not be valid. If an interview tool is said to be valid, it measures what it is supposed to measure—the potential productivity of a prospective employee. With regard to the effectiveness of the interview process, prevailing concepts include:

- Attitudes and biases that influence the interview process.
- Negative information about the applicant is weighed more heavily than positive information.
- Decisions are often formed in the first few minutes of the interview.
- In the unstructured interview, significant variance in ratings of candidates is common.
- Improved consistency between raters occurs in the structured format.
- The structured interview is generally a better predictor of job performance and overall effectiveness than the unstructured format.
- Validity increases when there is a team approach to interviewing.
- The interviewer tends to do most of the talking in an unstructured interview.

Interview Strategies

Despite these limitations, the interview remains a common method used for selecting applicants for job positions. Some strategies can minimize these drawbacks:

- Use more than one person to interview the applicant.
- Develop and use the same structured interview for the same position.
- Assess decision-making ability using case simulation.
- Use the same cluster of scenarios for each job category.
- Interview job candidates more than once.
- Provide training in effective interviewing techniques (e.g., communication skills; planning, conducting, and controlling the interview).

Managers must be careful to avoid unlawful inquiries during the hiring interview. Federal legislation prohibits asking certain questions of any applicant.

Topic	Acceptable	Unacceptable
Age	Interviewer can ask applicants if they are between age 18 and 70.	Questions about specific age or birth date are unacceptable.
Gender/ Race	Information pertaining to race or color cannot be requested as conditions of employment.	Inquiring about gender or race is unacceptable.
Marital status	Interviewer may inquire if applicant can adhere to work schedules within the context of other commitments.	Any questions about marital status, pregnancy, or children are prohibited.
Residence	It is acceptable to inquire about current address and length of residency.	It is unacceptable to ask about former addresses, who lives there, or if the applicant owns or rents.
Religion	Avoid discussion regarding religious beliefs or practices.	All questions about religion are prohibited unless the organization has a religious affiliation. Then, it is both appropriate and legal to verify information about the person's willingness to support the organization's values.
National Origin	Interviewer may inquire about languages the applicant is able to speak and/or read/write.	Cannot inquire about native birthplace or language.
Education	All inquiries about academic, vocational, and professional activities are appropriate, including schools attended.	Cannot ask about specific dates of educational experiences or religious school affiliations.
Health	General questions about the applicant's ability to perform the job are acceptable.	Inquiries about specific disabilities are prohibited. Employer must be able to justify any questions regarding an applicant's mental or physical health.

Table adapted from: Marquis, B. L., and Huston, C. J. (2002). *Leadership roles and management functions in nursing: Theory and application* (4th ed.). Philadelphia: Lippincott Williams & Wilkins.

Management Functions in Indoctrination

Indoctrination refers to the adjustment phase for a new employee. As a management function, indoctrination is planned and guided to help the employee adjust to the organization and work environment. The process instills a sense of belonging and improves productivity, reduces turnover, and enhances job satisfaction. The indoctrination process involves four components:

Induction: The first phase of indoctrination focuses on educating the employee about the institution and personnel policies (e.g., employee handbook).

Orientation: Provides more specific information about the job position and is usually conducted by the staff development department. The new employee is oriented to specific departments, such as dietary and pharmacy, as well as the individual nursing unit. Orientation includes reviewing unit policies, scheduling/staffing policies, and work assignment procedures.

Socialization: Different from orientation in that it involves the sharing of values and attitudes of the organization. During this phase of indoctrination, the employee is introduced to the culture of the organization and unit. A primary role of the unit leader/manager is the socialization process that is essential to the morale and enthusiasm of the new employee. It is during this phase that the employee develops a sense of the organization's value system (e.g., team approach).

Professional development: The nurse manager who fosters an environment of professionalism and values, supports growth, inquiry, and critical thinking will realize the benefits of higher-level nursing practice. Continuing education, competency-based training, mentorship, cross-training activities, and other formal and informal learning opportunities are ways to improve the contributions of the staff.

The Work Environment

The work environment is relevant to all levels of staff and affects job satisfaction. A successful work environment will depend on how comfortable the staff feels in the environment, the acceptance of new ideas and staff involvement, support that staff members receive for taking risks, clear and consistent communication, trust, the planning process and results, goals and objectives that are agreed upon and implemented, and the value that is placed on each employee.

Motivation

Motivation, or an internal desire to act, is closely related to empowerment. It is unique to each person. Clearly, motivated staff members are easier to work with and are more successful. Unmotivated staff members do just enough to get by, which affects staff morale. Typically, factors that influence motivation are pay/compensation, benefits, employee needs/abilities/ goals, the job that is to be done, management and leadership styles, and the interest, belonging, and commitment that the staff member has in the organization and the job itself.

Strategies to Develop and Support Motivation
- Be aware of the staff member's needs, goals, personal style, and situation.
- Identify mutual goals.
- Encourage self-determination.
- Reward positive attitude and desired behaviors.

- Communicate directly, openly, and honestly.
- Support mentorship and persons that serve as role models to others.
- Acknowledge persons with the desire to make a difference.
- Promote an environment of growth, caring, and commitment.

There are many theories that have been developed to explain motivation, yet there is no one accepted theory:

Maslow's Hierarchy of Needs: This theory identifies five basic hierarchical needs (physiological, safety, love, esteem, and self-actualization) as the basis of motivation. Success at each level, beginning with physiological and progressing to safety, love, esteem, and self-actualization, leads the person to the next level. Self-actualization, the final level of this theory, involves feelings of accomplishment and opportunities for growth, but is not always reached.

Alderfer's Modified-Need Hierarchy Theory: This theory is similar to Maslow's, but it emphasizes three levels of needs (existence needs, relatedness needs, and growth needs).

Argyris's Psychological Energy Theory: This theory focuses on the individual's goals. The more these goals are in tune with the organization's goals, the more the staff member will be motivated.

McClelland's Basic Needs Theory: This theory focuses on three basic needs that motivate people: achievement, power, and affiliation. If work responsibilities are matched with these needs, then staff will be more motivated.

Herzberg's Motivation-Hygiene Theory: This theory emphasizes the need for achievement, growth, responsibility, advancement, recognition, and the job itself. Dissatisfaction with work occurs when the employee thinks he/she is treated unfairly—in pay, benefits, job security, and supervision. These are "hygiene factors" that do not motivate, that create discontent, and do not make work more interesting. If a job is interesting, hygiene factors are better tolerated.

McGregor's Theory X and Theory Y: Theory X supports the assumption that people avoid work because they dislike it and are unmotivated. This results in the need for managers to use direction and control, leading to management that is far from positive. Staff members really want security. Theory Y makes the opposite assumption: people like work and are self-directed. According to Theory Y, work itself is rewarding; therefore, the management style that uses positive feedback and encourages staff participation and creativity will be more successful.

Skinner's Positive Reinforcement Theory (Behavior Modification): Skinner's theory focuses on behavior and the use of positive reinforcement to affect behavior. Providing positive feedback when work is successful is important. Negative feedback may decrease inadequate work, but it will not teach new behavior.

By using knowledge of these theories, managers can motivate staff by helping them gain strength and use their own inner motivation.

Empowerment

The process of sharing power and control for decisions contributes to employee generativity and job satisfaction. Individuals who possess the authority, responsibility, and freedom to act in a way that supports their own beliefs and goals are likely to experience more role contentment. Empowerment instills confidence in people and in their ability to succeed, which leads to higher quality performance in job-related activities. Empowered employees are likely to be more satisfied, and as such, employers enjoy the benefits of a self-motivated staff that is more likely to share in decision-making and problem-solving roles. This is likely to translate into increased productivity and reduced staff turnover and absenteeism. Staff participation in activities such as quality improvement, peer recognition programs, enrichment, and shared governance can contribute to an employee's professional growth and sense of empowerment. Concerns regarding lack of autonomy, insufficient time to perform required functions, or inability to access the necessary resources to provide professional services in a sufficient manner can be overcome through empowerment strategies. The leadership style of the nurse manager is key to the development of an empowered staff. The nurse manager who supports staff and offers opportunity for personal and professional growth is likely to create an environment in which nurses report greater role satisfaction.

Reality Shock

As the new graduate experiences clinical practice in the health care setting, some incongruence between the idealized concepts and actual practice may cause feelings of discouragement and disappointment. The shift from a setting where instructors maintained responsibility and control for the student's activities and decisions to a setting in which the nurse is autonomous and liable for own practice is one source of fear in the new graduate. Faced with unrealized expectations for the fantasized practice situation and potential lack of support, the new graduate is at risk for reality shock.

The health care environment today may contribute to the development of reality shock in the new graduate nurse. Job-related stress with little support for new graduates attempting to "get over the hurdle" and develop a more secure perspective acts as a deterrent for students. Many experienced staff members lack the initiative and energy to support the new graduate through this time. A mentoring relationship can foster an attitude of "I can do it" and provide insight into the daily practice situations likely to be encountered. Those experiencing disillusionment are at risk for burnout and reduced longevity in the practice setting.

Burnout

Burnout is a stress reaction that occurs when an employee experiences a state of role frustration, emotional exhaustion, depersonalization, and ineffective performance. This mental, emotional, and physical fatigue may be related to a sense of powerlessness. Chronic stress usually leads to a feeling of overload and eventually burnout.

Characteristics of Burnout

- Physical illness, stress-related disorders, such as chronic back pain, headaches, hypertension, ulcer disease, colitis, chronic fatigue or insomnia.
- Substance abuse, including alcohol, tobacco, or illicit drug use is common in people who are excessively stressed.
- Mental symptoms are evidenced by feelings of dread, negativism, depression, anxiety, and forgetfulness.
- Emotional responses are passivity, apathy, cynicism, anger and resentment, excessive worrying, and low self-esteem. Interpersonal conflicts are common with family, friends, and co-workers.
- Work-based effects include: low staff morale, alienation, decreased participation in unit- based activities, errors, poor decision-making, impaired problem-solving skills, absenteeism, sloppy penmanship, poor grooming, and termination.

Factors Contributing to Burnout
- Unrealistic workload
- Long hours
- Lack of control over schedule
- Feelings of powerlessness and lack of change related to actions
- Poor communication patterns within/between staff and leadership
- Lack of opportunity for advancement
- Limited decision-making opportunities
- Low level of appreciation for efforts and contributions
- Insufficient salary to meet needs
- Unsupportive management team

Burnout Prevention Strategies
The most important strategies to prevent burnout should be directed toward supporting, encouraging, and valuing staff and their contributions to the function of the team. A few of the ways that a nurse manager could enhance the staff's job satisfaction may include:
- Involving staff in planning activities and practice-based decision-making
- Providing educational opportunities for professional growth
- Understanding the needs of the staff and empathizing with stress experiences
- Actively listening to staff concerns and taking action to rectify the situation if possible
- Offering programs for stress management to staff
- Being available to staff
- Conducting performance appraisals in a timely manner using appropriate feedback
- Allowing participatory scheduling as appropriate for the practice setting
- Mentoring, encouraging, and supporting staff in their professional role
- Providing coffee breaks and meal breaks away from the work unit

Much of what is discussed in this module, if done correctly, will help to prevent burnout. Other strategies to prevent burnout include:
- Planning that includes staff involvement
- Providing educational opportunities
- Managers who understand stress and the needs of the staff
- Managers who make themselves available to their staff members
- Appropriate scheduling and staffing levels for client needs
- Performance appraisals that occur more often than annually and provide positive feedback when the employee excels and guidance when the employee needs it
- Stress management programs
- Encouraging staff members to recognize the importance of their personal life

To help prevent burnout, organizations may provide childcare, exercise classes, membership to gyms, and other benefits to assist staff in caring for themselves and their families.

Conflict Management

Conflict is the result of opposing thoughts, ideas, feelings, perceptions, behaviors, values, opinions, or actions. It is an inevitable part of professional, social, and personal life, and can result in constructive or destructive consequences. In some regards, conflict can be the stimulant for growth; open and honest communication may occur in the process of dealing with conflict. Conflict that is handled positively as controversy, instead of a dispute, may yield benefit to the group by increasing group cohesion and commitment to common goals, facilitating understanding, promoting problem-solving, motivating the group to change, and stimulating creativity. Negative consequences of conflict can produce divisiveness, rivalry and competition, misperceptions, distrust, frustration, and dissatisfaction with the outcome.

There are three broad types of conflict:

Intrapersonal conflict occurs within an individual in situations involving a choice between mutually exclusive alternatives. The perceived incompatibility in ideas, ethical standards, or course of action can result in intrapersonal struggle. This internal tension often occurs as a conflict in roles or situational impossibility. In the health care setting, a nurse may experience intrapersonal conflict when providing care to an anxious client who needs time and support; while at the same time, the nurse needs to complete other job-related tasks. Other examples of intrapersonal conflict would be the nurse who is undecided about attending a continuing education conference or is worried about working overtime due to staffing pressures. The nurse manager may be faced with this type of conflict when confronting a staff member who is also a personal friend with a performance-related complaint.

Interpersonal conflict involves two or more persons who do not share the same perspective, views, or attitude in a given situation. A disagreement between nurses, clients, family members, and within a health care team can result in dispute or growth. Issues relating to diversity in lifestyle, values, and ideas are usually the source of dispute between or among persons. For example, a nurse working on a general medical unit might express frustration because of an issue related to mandatory overtime. Issues of fairness can generate feelings of interpersonal conflict.

Intragroup or organizational conflict exists between two or more persons within a group or organization. Issues related to policies, norms and expectations for behaviors, role, communication, and authority are often sources of organizational conflict. New systems may stimulate misunderstanding or debate. Change in leadership is another source of disharmony within a group expecting to achieve a common goal. A practical example of this in the health care setting would be if the nurse and social worker serving on a multidisciplinary team at a public health department have a disagreement about who should take the primary role in follow-up care in the community setting. Intragroup conflict may occur in a team of nurses functioning in a shared-governance model when the person who has the responsibility for devising a specific unit-based protocol is not clearly identified.

Conflict is inevitable, but it can have positive outcomes and can be approached in a variety of ways. The approach depends upon the specific type of conflict, but the optimal goal of any approach is creating a win-win solution for all involved. The manager's primary role is to identify the most appropriate strategy for conflict management. The negotiation for conflict resolution requires effective management and leadership skills. Although successful negotiation often requires risk taking, managers must be well prepared, armed with self-confidence, multiple alternatives, and a clear bottom line.

Strategies for Conflict Management

Conflict Management Strategy	Type	Operational Definition
Win-Lose Strategies	Competing	One party seeks to win, regardless of the cost to the others involved. This type of win-lose conflict resolution leaves the losing party angry and frustrated and is used by managers only when a quick or unpopular decision needs to be made.
	Compromising	Compromise is often seen as a 'win-lose' strategy since each person gives up something. It is appropriate, however, when an agreement is needed and the goals of both parties are at odds. Compromising can be a potential lose-lose strategy when either or both parties perceive they have given up more than the other; therefore, both parties must agree upon relinquishing something of equal value in order for this strategy to be effective.
Lose-Win Strategies	Accommodating	One party sacrifices a belief or goal, wanting the other party to win.
Lose-Lose Strategies	Avoiding or Withdrawing	Both parties are aware of the conflict, but choose not to acknowledge it and/or attempt to resolve the conflict.
	Smoothing or Suppressing	An approach where one party tries to reduce emotions without addressing the problem itself. It is often used to preserve or maintain a peaceful work environment, but involves sacrificing personal goals or values; however, the problem still exists.
Win-Win Strategies	Collaborating	A cooperative approach where both parties work together to establish a common goal.

Let's look at an example and demonstrate how several of these types of strategies might apply to a given situation. An experienced nurse on a urology unit arrives to work on the night shift. The unit manager immediately asks the nurse to float to a pediatrics unit because the hospital census is high and they are understaffed. The nurse has always maintained a positive attitude when asked to float to medical-surgical units but states she does not feel comfortable in the pediatric setting. The manager insists the nurse is the most qualified. Let's analyze this situation from the nurse's point of view.

Competing: If the nurse truly feels unqualified to float to pediatrics then this approach may be appropriate–the nurse must win and the manager must lose. Although risking termination by refusing the float, the nurse should take an assertive approach and inform the manager that children would be placed at risk.

Accommodating: If the nurse decides to accommodate the manager's request, then the children may be at risk for incompetent care. Practice liability is another issue for consideration.

Avoiding or Suppressing: The nurse basically cannot use this strategy since the manager has the power. The conflict cannot be simply avoided; the nurse cannot withdraw from the situation without some sort of negative consequence.

Compromising: This approach generally minimizes the losses for all involved while making certain each party gains something. In this case, the nurse might negotiate a compromise. For example, the nurse might offer to float to another medical-surgical unit if someone from that unit feels comfortable in the pediatric environment. Although each party is giving up something, (e.g., the manager gives in to a different solution and the nurse still has to float), this sort of compromise can result in a win-win resolution.

Collaboration: Ideally, this approach is preferred for conflict management since it results in a win-win situation. If the nurse and manager can identify an agreeable goal and work together to find alternative solutions, then the best results can occur for everyone. In this situation, perhaps the pediatric nurse manager could join in the problem-solving process. Although this strategy is ideal, it is not always realistic given time constraints in certain situations. It may be that compromise is the most appropriate choice for this situation.

Performance Appraisal

Performance appraisal is used in the evaluation process for nursing employees to assess the effectiveness and efficiency of care delivered to clients. It is a formal, systematic, and standardized evaluation process that provides the employee with a measure of perceived value of his/her contributions and quality of work. This mechanism opens lines of communication between the nurse manager and staff member, whereby problematic issues can be discussed or recognition and praise can be offered. This method of outcomes-based feedback is defined by the specific position description and standards of practice within that role. Performance, as a result of skills, knowledge, interpersonal style and motivation, is considered. In this setting, the two parties usually discuss professional goals and steps to achieve that outcome. Peer evaluation and self-report may be included in the performance appraisal process.

Process of Performance Appraisal

The nurse manager needs to be prepared for the evaluation of, as well as knowledgeable about, the position description, policies, and procedures. If the employee is a union member, then union contract policies and procedures must be adhered to during the entire process. The performance appraisal process is continuous. As soon as it is complete, it begins again when the employee identifies his/her goals for the next year. There is no doubt that it is time-consuming and requires careful documentation. It is critical that the manager avoid bias and preconceived notions about the employee that may act as barriers to open discussion and evaluation.

The steps in the performance appraisal process are:

Data collection: Evaluation requires accurate data about the employee's performance. Methods that may be used to collect these data are anecdotal notes that are kept by the manager throughout the year, observation, checklists and rating scales, continuing education attendance records, review of the employee's documentation in clients' medical records, incident reports, and quality improvement data.

Preparation: The performance appraisal interview is a key element for making the interview more successful and a positive experience for all involved. The interviewer must be knowledgeable about the position description, and have relevant data about the candidate, both positive and negative. The applicant should come prepared with a resume or professional Curriculum Vitae and copy of professional goals.

Conducting the appraisal: Privacy and time are critical. There should be no interruptions. The nurse performing the appraisal sets a tone for an open discussion. The interview appraisal needs to be documented immediately following it, and the employee should be given a copy of the evaluation that is placed in the employee's personnel file.

Follow-up: The manager needs to follow up with the employee. How is the employee doing? Are the goals set during the evaluation being met? If not, how can the manager assist the employee? In addition, the manager must complete organizational forms, such as forms for promotion, pay changes, etc.

Common Errors in Performance Evaluation

Although criteria such as job description and standards of care are used, performance evaluations are subjective and open to human judgment and influenced by internal and external factors. The unit manager should be aware of several common errors involving evaluation.

Halo Error results when the evaluator allows one trait to influence evaluation of other characteristics. For example, a nurse with an excellent attendance record consistently works overtime to complete the assignments. The unit manager gives the nurse a good rating, allowing excellent attendance and punctuality to offset mediocre time management. In addition, evaluators are likely to rate an employee higher or lower than deserved, based on identification of deficiencies similar to the evaluator's own shortcomings.

Horns Error is essentially the opposite of the halo error and occurs when the evaluator is overly critical. The following are some examples of the horns error.

- Rating the employee lower based on a mistake made in the past
- Ranking personnel negatively based on personality trait(s) rather than work performance
- Ranking the employee's job performance lower than deserved based on the evaluator's unfamiliarity with the job
- Allowing an entire work group to negatively influence the evaluation of a particular individual in the group

Contrast Error occurs when the evaluator rates the employee opposite from the way they perceive their own abilities and traits. For example, a manager who believes her personal time management skills are excellent may score the nurse lower on time management even without supportive evidence.

Recency Error is the tendency to base the performance appraisal on recent events rather than on performance over the entire evaluation period.

Central Tendency Error occurs when the evaluator is reluctant to give a true appraisal, rating all employees as average. This is also called leniency error and is often the result of the evaluator's desire to be liked by all employees.

How to Avoid Common Errors

It is essential that the manager use strategies that increase fairness and accuracy in the evaluation process. Attitudes and biases of interviewers and evaluators cannot be eliminated entirely. However, steps can be taken to reduce subjectivity and common errors discussed above. Probably the most important step is for the appraiser to be aware of personal biases. When the appraiser believes personal bias is influencing the evaluation, another manager should be consulted.

- Data collection should be done systematically and regularly throughout the evaluation period to reduce recency error. In addition, it is essential that the manager focus on job performance rather than personality, and document specific events or activities at the time they occur to avoid perception and gaps in recall of the actual details.

- Traditional rating scales highlight personal characteristics or traits and are subject to halo and horns effect as well as central tendency. Many health care institutions have adopted behavior-oriented performance appraisal systems rather than using tools that evaluate traits (e.g., dependability and initiative), which are difficult to measure and may cause legal problems.

- Although checklists offer a variety of job-related behaviors with reduced subjectivity inherent in trait-rating scales, the checklist approach falls short because it often does not incorporate performance standards.

- Forced-distribution techniques can be used to reduce errors of central tendency by forcing the evaluator to choose statements that best and least describe the person. The evaluator does not know the scoring method; therefore, bias is reduced.

The Performance Appraisal Interview

The performance interview provides the venue for mutual exchange of information between the employee and the employer. Both parties can determine if the qualifications, professional goals, employment situation, environment, roles, and responsibilities are a good match. A collaborative approach for goal setting and future professional activities for growth is critical for future performance and role satisfaction. Strategies that a nurse manager may use to facilitate a positive environment for the interview may include:

- Conducting the interview in a quiet, private room that is free of interruptions.

- Maintaining an open and relaxed posture to convey feeling of receptivity.

- Encouraging active participation in the goal-setting, and problem-solving processes.

- Allowing the employee to express opinions, concerns, and questions regarding the appraisal process and any other job or role-related function, orally or in writing.

- Discussing both positive and negative performance issues honestly and accurately, including specific details. Be constructive in the feedback for the employee.

- Offering an opportunity to generate a mutual plan for action and documenting it in the employee file.
- Determining follow-up as needed.

Discipline

The employee whose performance does not meet the expectations will require disciplinary action. Experiences in discipline are difficult for the managers and staff who are involved. How the issue is handled depends upon the policies and procedures for this occurrence. If the organization is unionized, the union will be actively involved in this process. To prevent disciplinary problems, the organization's policies and procedures need to be understood by all staff members to whom they apply.

Before a disciplinary action is taken, it is very important for the manager to investigate the incident or situation carefully. When the manager meets with the employee, privacy is critical. Rules are applied consistently, allowing the employee to have the opportunity to discuss the issue and his/her viewpoint. The manager needs to listen to the employee's side, as new information may be obtained, and consider the employee's past history—performance, attitude, work record related to attendance, etc. When action is taken, it needs to be clear to the employee. The nurse manager clearly and objectively documents the incident, pattern of behavior, or outcome-based performance. Follow-up is crucial and detailed feedback must be given to the employee. Accurate documentation in the employee's record is absolutely necessary.

Progressive Discipline

The need for progressive discipline occurs when the employee's behavior or performance continues to fall below standards. When behavioral or performance problems are not resolved with coaching, the manager has formal authority and responsibility to take progressively stronger forms of discipline to correct the action. Most progressive disciplinary processes involve four steps:

- **Step 1**: Counsel the employee about job performance and be specific about what the expectations are for improvement.
- **Step 2**: Give the employee an oral and written reprimand that includes an explanation of the incident(s), a plan of action, and the employee's perspective and opinion of the plan. An oral reprimand alone is of limited value; it would be difficult to prove that a warning was given. The employee must sign the document. The employee's signature does not convey agreement but simply means the individual has read the documentation and is aware of the problem.
- **Step 3**: If unacceptable behavior or performance persists, the next progressive step is suspension. The individual is informed that he/she is not to return to work for a specified period. This conveys to the employee the critical nature of the behavior, and hopefully prompts serious attention to the problem. After the suspension period, the employee is permitted to return to work.
- **Step 4**: If the employee's behavior continues, the final step is termination. Individuals may voluntarily end their employment at some time during the disciplinary process.

Two problems commonly occur during the disciplinary process. The first of these is the inclination to wait until emotions are high and then the manager overreacts. The second problem occurs because the manager wants the relationship to end on a positive note, and therefore, the terminal evaluation is overly complementary even in the face of unsatisfactory job performance. This discredits the manager's previous evaluation and may result in a liability problem should the former employee decide to pursue legal action.

During progressive discipline, the manager should adhere to the general principles of performance appraisal (e.g., data gathering, documentation, etc.). Investigate the situation thoroughly, asking these questions:

- Has the employee been involved in a similar situation before?
- Was she/he disciplined for this behavior?
- How did he/she respond to corrective action?
- How serious or potentially serious is the current problem?
- Who else was involved?
- Does the employee have a history of other disciplinary problems?
- What is the quality of the employee's work?
- Have other employees experienced the same problem?
- Were there factors that could have contributed to the problem?
- What disciplinary action is suggested by organizational policy?
- Will the suggested disciplinary action prevent the problem from recurring?

Documentation of critical incidents and anecdotal notes must be collected throughout the employee's counseling sessions and evaluation process. When cases go to an appeal board, the burden of proof is on the employer to prove that the employee's behavior and/or job performance clearly warranted disciplinary action. It is worth noting again that clear and accurate documentation is essential. Those in attendance, including the employee, should sign a record of the conference discussion. A copy should be personally delivered to the employee. The conduct that is being criticized must not have been ignored or condoned at an earlier time. Unacceptable behavior is being excused when it is not dealt with in an open and timely manner. One of the most difficult tasks for a manager is ensuring that all employees with similar problems have received similar consequences. A third person should be present to validate what occurs if the manager anticipates that a disciplinary conference will be problematic. The employee has a right to know that another person will be present and the employee has the right to bring an individual to represent his/her own interests.

When using progressive discipline, the steps are sequential for violations of the same rule. Although the discipline process should be progressive, immediate suspension or dismissal may be necessary if the behavior causes a serious problem, such as potential client injury. The manager needs to avoid holding resolved transgressions against the employee and future performance appraisals are to be as objective as the employee's first evaluation.

Most employment manuals list actions/behaviors that are grounds for immediate dismissal. It is also important to note that many states have a "dismissal without cause law." Unions may specify in contracts that firing without cause and the specific grounds for immediate dismissal be outlined.

Suggestions for the Disciplinary Conference

- Clearly state the problem, referring to previous counseling sessions. Managers have the authority by definition of their role and need to avoid being apologetic.

- Ask the employee why improvement has not occurred. This allows the employee to give his/her perspective, discuss any factors unknown to the manager, and conveys to the employee a sense of fairness.

- Explain the disciplinary action planned. The employee should be very clear about the reason and nature of disciplinary action because it should have been explained during the last conference. It is important to summarize 'why' the specific disciplinary action is necessary.

- Describe the expected behavioral change. Employees having performance or behavior problems often require direction. The steps needed to achieve the change should be given, along with an explanation of the consequences of failure to change. Clarity is essential so that the employee is not confused about the seriousness of the consequences and is aware that follow-up will occur.

- Get acceptance of the plan. The manager should give support and convey an interest in the employee's personal growth. This helps the employee see that the discipline is directed at the behavior rather than the individual. Again, care must be taken to avoid giving confusing messages while giving support and counsel.

- Share documentation. The employee should receive a copy of the disciplinary action form.

The Grievance Process

The manager can reduce risk of being involved in a grievance by fostering a work environment that emphasizes clear communication and fair, constructive discipline. When conflicts or disagreements between employees and management do occur, they can usually be reconciled informally through communication and negotiation. However, a formal grievance procedure should be available to employees any time they perceive they have been unfairly treated by management.

The steps of the formal grievance process are generally outlined in union contracts or administrative policy and procedure manuals:

- Formally present complaint(s) using the proper chain of command.

- If resolution does not occur at some level, a formal hearing is held.

- If differences cannot be settled through this process, the matter may be resolved in a process known as arbitration, where both sides agree on the selection of a professional mediator who reviews the grievance, finalizes data gathering, and interviews those involved prior to coming to a decision.

The goal of the process is not to win, but to reach a satisfactory outcome for both the employee and the organization. Both parties must be open to discussion and negotiation.

Termination

Termination may be voluntary or involuntary. Involuntary termination of employment should occur only after progressive discipline and notification of performance problems. Organization policies and procedures must be followed during this process. Documentation is absolutely essential. If the employee involved is a member of the union, then all procedures established by the union contract must be strictly followed. Managers need to follow rules consistently and not convey favor of some employees over others. In the voluntary termination situation, there is a "letting go" experience as the staff member prepares to leave, whereby the person withdraws emotionally. Production may also decrease during this phase.

Those who leave involuntarily are more difficult to deal with and may cause other staff to be concerned for the loss of their jobs. Involuntary termination is likely to cause the employee to experience many feelings, such as loss, anger, sadness, and confusion. Some employees who leave involuntarily may be destructive to the group function, cohesiveness, and productivity. Some organizations prefer that the person leave quickly, rather than have a long, drawn-out period before the termination date. Terminated employees usually require information from Human Resources about their pay, benefits, and references.

Turnover

Turnover is costly for health care organizations. If the turnover level is high, the organization needs to analyze the reasons for the turnover and take preventive action. Many organizations have a termination interview that is used to collect data about the reasons staff leave voluntarily. Frequent reasons that are given are:

- Lack of staff empowerment, autonomy, and respect
- Poor staff communication
- Poor staff-management communication
- Inadequate compensation
- Inadequate benefits
- Scheduling issues
- Inability to work with immediate supervisor
- Inadequate staff education or support for further education
- Lack of opportunities for advancement
- Non-nursing tasks done by nurses
- Lack of nursing leadership

Studies have shown that employees are reluctant to be totally truthful in a termination or exit interview. They tend to minimize their reasons for leaving or make safe responses for fear of the negative consequences of an honest response. Employees who quit may "play it safe" and simply state that they have found a better opportunity, regardless of the actual reason for electing termination.

Labor Relations

Many health care organizations have union contracts for at least some of their employees. Managers who hire and terminate employees cannot be members of the union. Each union contract is unique, so it is impossible to discuss the details of the contracts. It is critical for management to understand the contract and managerial responsibilities. Critical issues in labor relations are discipline, hiring, termination, benefits and salary, and scheduling in terms of the employment agreement. Collective bargaining joins employees together so that they can act as one to obtain benefits, salary, and the working conditions that they believe they need. Employees pay a union membership fee. There is a complicated process for the election of a labor contract, and there are laws about collective bargaining conduct. Collective bargaining is the mechanism for settling labor disputes with negotiation.

Critical Thinking Exercise: Human Resource Management

1. As a team leader, you focus on the following needs of your team members. What motivation theory would apply to each of these approaches?

    a. People need to work.

    b. Self-actualization is the highest need.

    c. You match work assignments to a staff member's need for achievement, power, and affiliation.

2. What criteria would you use to determine your own satisfaction with your job?

3. You are a nurse manager for an emergency department. One of the nurses has called in sick three times in the last pay period, which is unusual for this nurse. You are auditing the medical records and notice that this same nurse has made several important errors in the past month in her documentation. You decide that you need to speak with her, but as you leave your office you overhear this nurse in the treatment area complaining about the level of work and the awful work environment in the ED. What might this nurse be experiencing and how might you approach her about her absenteeism, errors, and what you've overheard?

4. What can be done to prevent other staff from experiencing discontentment with the level of work or work environment?

5. Your next task that day is to review requests from your staff to attend several continuing education seminars. They are requesting paid time off for attending. What criteria might you use to evaluate the seminars?

6. It is time for performance appraisals for two nurses and one UAP working in the unit. Discuss the process you will use to complete these evaluations.

7. Effective mentoring of women has become more prevalent in the workforce over the past 20 years.

    a.   As a novice nurse, what are the advantages of being mentored by an experienced nurse?

    b.   What are the characteristics of effective nurse mentoring?

CHAPTER 9

Time Management

Key Points

- Time management is an ongoing process of clarifying vision and values, identifying goals, and organizing a plan of action.
- Time management directly effects efficiency and effectiveness.
- All nurses need to use time management.
- The first step is to diagnose time management problems and then change the behavior to achieve the goal.

Overview

Time is a valuable resource in the work environment, but there seems to be less and less of it. Perceived excessive demands coupled with an ability to achieve the goals in the given time is a major cause of stress for all workers in the health care environment, which can impair their desire to care for clients. Learning to manage time is critical for all staff and managers and it is a skill that must be renewed, as it is easy to slip back into a situation where time is lost and stress increases.

Why Is Time Management Important?

Time management directly affects work efficiency and effectiveness. Most people have to make a conscious effort to learn how to manage their time and practice this skill. Time management affects quality of care, use of resources (people, budget, supplies, equipment), organizational culture, responsiveness to consumers/customers, team collaboration, communication, decision- making, and planning. Everything is affected by time and the ability to manage it.

Diagnosis: What Are Your Time Management Issues?

Without knowing what a problem is, it cannot be solved. Make a list of your specific problems. Some common problems include getting started and sticking to a project, organizing your day, procrastinating, inability to set limits, losing information, being interrupted, overworking, leaving work on time—and more. Three principles to help you get started are:

- Establish long-term and short-term goals
- Set priorities
- Stay focused to achieve goals

Taking Action

Setting Goals and Prioritizing

- Identify what needs to be done and establish goals.

- Prioritize by considering your overall goals, the urgency or deadline, if it needs to be delegated, and how one activity relates to another. For example, does one activity need to be done before another?

- Set priority client outcomes based on the urgency of each client's needs. For example, nurses in the emergency department see first-priority urgent clients immediately, second- priority urgent clients as soon as possible, and third-priority non-urgent clients after the most urgent cases receive emergency care.

- Set priorities related to what you like to do and what you want to avoid. Sometimes you cannot avoid the task, and this will affect your priorities.

- Review your priorities and your goals, ensuring that there is no conflict.

Achieving Your Goals: Strategies

- Delegate tasks to help get the job done: the right person for the right job at the right time.

- Effective scheduling of work, while keeping schedule flexible.

- Provide time to deal with unforeseen interruptions or opportunities that may arise on a daily basis.

- Avoid wasting time by considering the biggest time wasters (e.g., postponing action, not having a quiet place to work, socializing with others, doing other staff members' work, working on low-priority projects first, interfering with others' work.) You can be your own worst interrupter.

- If your goals are not reasonable or clear, achieving them will be difficult.

- Waiting for the "right time to do something" often leads to failure to do it. This is procrastination.

- Use a "to-do" list and check off the items completed to give yourself a boost.

- Consider the routine tasks that must be done daily, and then the other tasks that must done. Screen your items and prioritize. For some tasks it may be best to delegate them to others. Consider what will happen if you do not do the task, or if you do a scaled-down version. Is the task worth the time required to do it?

- Leave some time for creative work.

- Use problem solving and critical thinking to "think outside the box."

- Prepare for meetings, but before you schedule them, think about the best way to deal with the various issues: could you use mail, fax, or make a telephone call? Which would be better–an individual or group meeting, etc?

- Reading is important, but it needs to be done efficiently. Try to do this by scanning the table of contents; read only what you need; keep a file of articles you want to read when time allows. If you find yourself reading something that is not relevant, stop reading.

- Set up a time in your schedule to read correspondence. A helpful approach is to never read something twice if you can help it. Act on it after reading it so that you do not have to reread it. There are some items that are more complex and require additional reading, but this is not the major portion of most correspondence.

- Telephone calls can consume time planned for other endeavors. You might set aside a time to return calls. Keep telephone numbers available. Limit the length of calls. Save difficult calls for when you have privacy and time. Prepare for complex calls to decrease their length. When you leave a message, recommend a time to return the call. Voice mail may take care of the need for a return call. Use mail to cut down on telephone calls that might get you more involved than is helpful.

- It is important to praise yourself when tasks are completed and even reward yourself. Do not forget to take some breaks—refresh yourself.

Questions to Ask Yourself

- At the end of the day, what do I hope to have accomplished?
- What task am I most concerned about getting done?
- What needs to be done next?
- What will happen if I don't get this done?

Time Savers

- The major time waster is not being able to find information when you need it. Develop a system that works for you so that information can be accessed readily.
- Arrange materials and supplies in an orderly fashion.
- Learn to say "no" graciously and with confidence.
- Make use of idle time: what to do when waiting for a telephone call, an appointment, etc.
- Build in a time cushion. Tasks always seem to take longer than you think.
- Make quick decisions on small matters (decisions take energy).
- When you can, do two things at once (except when directly dealing with a client, family, or staff member).
- Keep a list of "fill-in" jobs or five-minute tasks that can be done quickly when you have spare time. Accomplishing these tasks will make you feel like you are moving ahead.
- Minimize distractions and interruptions.
- Set a deadline and adhere to it.

Critical Thinking Exercise: Time Management

1. What time management issues do you have?

2. How might you resolve these problems?

CHAPTER 10

Delegation

Key Points

- Delegation involves empowering others to perform a task or assume a role for the shared goal of the group.
- Three factors impact the delegation process:
  - Responsibility is the obligation to perform a given task or function.
  - Authority refers to the decision-making power.
  - Accountability relates to the acceptance of responsibility for the outcome of a duty.
- Delegation process involves:
  - Identification of the need
  - Selection of the most suitable person to perform the duty
  - Clear communication of expectations
  - Acceptance of the task
  - Monitoring of performance (periodic inspection)
  - Feedback
- Imprudent delegation can result in liability issues. Appropriate selection and monitoring of performance is essential.

Overview

Delegation is an act to enhance the efficiency and effectiveness of managerial or clinical nursing practice. It involves empowering another to perform a task or function in a specified role for the common goal of the group. Delegation does not imply an abdication of responsibility but instead will result in affecting a multiplicity of efforts. The assignment of responsibility to a competent person who is equipped to perform the duty can increase productivity and job satisfaction. However, delegation does entail organization and supervision to maintain safety and quality in the practice setting. Although the person delegating maintains the ultimate authority and ultimate responsibility for the task, all persons involved on both ends (delegation and acceptance) assume accountability for the action. Clear expression of goals and expectations is key to achieving the desired outcome. Mutual satisfaction is more likely when both parties understand the need for the task, the way it will be carried out, timeline for completion, and beneficial effect that will likely occur as a result of the action. Accountability for the outcome of the task remains the responsibility of the manager.

Benefits of Delegation

- Saves time
- Increases productivity and multiplicity of efforts
- More staff involvement leads to ownership of ideas and shared goals
- Increases job satisfaction
- Boosts self-esteem and confidence
- More group cohesion
- Increases management skills
- Identifies, early on, future leaders and managers

Considerations for Selection of Appointee

- Education
- Skills, training, and experience
- Potential for harm
- Complexity of the task
- Level of critical thinking required to complete task
- Ability to communicate with others as it pertains to the duty
- Demonstrated competence
- Agency policies and procedures
- Licensing legislation (State Nurse Practice Acts)

Effective Ways to Delegate

- Identify and communicate the need for the task to be performed.
- Select the right person for the job; consider who is best matched, qualified, willing, and able.
- Consider what other responsibilities and demands on time the appointee has.
- Determine the resources and information necessary to tackle the project or function in the role.
- Carefully explain the details of the assignment. Encourage the person to ask questions to clarify any uncertainties.
- Empower this person with the authority necessary to perform the function. Convey confidence in the appointee's abilities.
- Set a realistic time frame for completion of the task. Check regularly to ascertain if problems are preventing achievement of the goal.
- Express appreciation for saving time. A thank you goes a long way in facilitating team spirit and future cooperation.

Barriers to Effective Delegation

- Choosing persons who lack the skills, education, training, or ability to perform the task
- Under-delegation, whereby the workload is not sufficiently reduced

- Delegation by default
- Poor timing
- Absence of supervision or monitoring
- Poor communication with unclear expectations, description of duty, or timeline for completion
- Excessive control
- Lack of trust or confidence in others
- "I can do it myself" attitude
- Lack of formal education in undergraduate curricula
- Insufficient continuing education and staff development offerings for practicing RNs

Delegation As It Applies to the Health Care Organization

- Selection of an appointee for the appointed task is determined in part by the defined position as stated. Modifications to position description may be necessary when expanding the scope of responsibilities and duties.
- Implementation of a delegated task or role involves conformity to the organizational policies and procedures.
- Staff development is an aid to enhance staff qualification and acceptance of the task.
- Incentive programs and formal feedback are necessary to encourage staff to participate in additional duties.

Health Care Organization Issues

- There must be conformation with policies and procedures.
- Position descriptions must be considered and updated as needs change.
- Staff education is used to prepare staff for delegation.
- Feedback and reward systems are necessary to encourage staff.
- State Nurse Practice Acts, which offer guidelines for delegation, should be available on all client care units.

Delegation Process

Identify and define what needs to be delegated: This requires that you are knowledgeable about the job/task/procedure and clearly understand the staff member's position description. You cannot ask a staff member to do something that is beyond the defined role, or something that he/she has not been trained to do. You must also assess the specific situation to determine if this is the correct time or situation to delegate a task. In general, you need to consider regulations and practice acts, standards, position descriptions, policies and procedures, organizational structure, and your resources.

Select the best person for the job/activity: Delegation requires that you consider all factors before making a decision, such as the acuity of the clients, resources available, the time factor, complexity, and priority of the task. Education and experience of the staff member, interest of the staff member, the amount of monitoring that will be required, and staff member's workload should also be considered.

Communicate the job/activity: Clear communication of the task is critical to success. Appropriate direction is reasonable, complete, clear, and, if detailed and complex, it should be in writing. The staff member needs to know what is to be done, to whom, when, time limits or limits on what the staff member may do, feedback required, and any other specific directions to complete the task.

Accept the delegated task: The staff member must accept the delegated task and indicate his/ her willingness and acceptance by asking questions if he/she is unclear about the responsibility.

Provide feedback and monitoring: Delegation does not mean assigning a task to a staff member and then forgetting about it. Monitoring and follow-up are required. The amount of monitoring will vary, depending on the task, the staff member, and the particular situation. Too much monitoring can be just as bad as too little. Staff also needs feedback. Let the collaborative team know that they have done something well, and if negative criticism is required, it should be done in private and should include both positive and negative feedback.

The Five Rights of Delegation

Right Task: Identify the appropriate delegation activities for specific clients and delegate appropriate activities to appropriate levels of team members (LPN, UAP, EMT, etc.)

Right Circumstance: Assess the health status and complexity of care required by clients and match the complexity of care demands to the skill level of the caregiver.

Right Person:
- Assess and verify the competency of the caregiver.
- Continually review the performance of team members relative to care competency.
- Assess team member performance based on standards and, when necessary, take steps to remediate failure to meet standards.

Right Direction/Communication: Communicate the following either in writing or orally:
- What data needs to be collected
- The method and timeline for reporting
- Specific activity(ies) to be performed; client-specific instructions
- Expected results, timelines and expectations for follow-up communication

Right Supervisor/Evaluation: The delegating nurse must:
- Provide supervision, either directly or indirectly (e.g., assigning supervision to another licensed nurse).
- Provide directions and understandable expectations of the activity(ies) to be performed
  - Monitor performance
  - Receive and provide feedback
  - Intervene if necessary
  - Assure clear documentation

- Review entire delegation process
  - Evaluate the client
  - Evaluate delegate's performance
  - Evaluate the activity being performed

Liability and Delegation

There is a risk of liability with delegation. The risk relates to the appropriateness of the delegation to an individual (skills and experience, position description, type of task, regulations and Nurse Practice Acts, policies and procedures, etc.) and the monitoring of the performance. Nurses need to use informed judgment when decisions are made regarding the delegation process.

Tasks That Can be Delegated by Registered Nurses

Under their direction, RNs may delegate the following duties to LPNs:
- Updating the initial RN assessment of a client
- Teaching a client from a standard care plan
- Initiating and maintaining intravenous lines, blood transfusions, hyperalimentation, and giving medications, including IV push and IV piggyback medications (in some states only)
- Removing sutures and inserting feeding tubes (in some states only)

Under their direction, RNs may delegate the following duties to unlicensed assistive personal (UAPs):
- Activities of daily living
- Bathing
- Grooming
- Dressing
- Toileting
- Ambulating
- Feeding
- Positioning
- Bedmaking
- Specimen collection
- Intake and output
- Vital signs

Critical Thinking Exercise: Delegation

1. Name three reasons why it might be important for you as a manager to delegate some of your responsibilities. What three tasks do you think you can delegate and why?

2. It is important to know yourself when you delegate. Take this time to honestly evaluate yourself and your use of delegation. Consider the purposes of delegation and the problems or disadvantages of using delegation.

3. You are asking an unlicensed assistive personnel (UAP) on the unit to assist you in the admission process for preoperative care. What factors would you consider as you delegate this task?

CHAPTER 11

Quality Improvement

Key Points

- Health care quality involves the pursuit of excellence in the delivery of care.
- Continuous quality improvement is instrumental in the identification of actual and potential problems as well as designing specific solutions.
- Continuous quality improvement programs are essential to accountability for professional practice.
- Quality monitoring activities are based on structure, process, and outcomes.
- The accreditation process is an outcomes-based evaluation that requires measurement of organizational goals and objectives.
- The national standards for Culturally and Linguistically Appropriate Services (CLAS) address the inequities in health care provision that effect ethnic groups and people of color.
- Case management approach is implemented for clients with complex health care to ensure that they receive appropriate care in an appropriate manner.
- Total quality management (TQM) is an organizational philosophy that is directed toward customer/client satisfaction.
- Continuous quality improvement (CQI) is a process involving a multidisciplinary team who analyzes the system (based on data collected), measures objective(s) and outcomes, and proposes informed changes.

Overview

Quality-monitoring activities have historically referred to quality assurance (QA) programs, which involve evaluating a system, process, or activity based on a previously established standard. This QA process focused on the detection of errors and inefficiencies through chart audit, incident reports, direct observation, and customized audit tools. The evaluation structure more commonly used today is continuous quality improvement (CQI), which is also outcome-based but focuses on strategies for positive change. This philosophy involves the members of the health care team to maintain quality and strive for improvement. CQI activities are closely tied to accountability issues. The institution's accreditation has far-reaching implications in terms of public perception, designation as a teaching facility, and qualification for federal monies through programs such as Medicare/Medicaid.

Aspects of Health Care Quality

A definition of health care quality might include such characteristics as appropriateness of care, timeliness, client satisfaction, effectiveness and efficiency, and safety. Three elements for evaluation are structure, process, and outcome(s). In the past, the primary focus was on the first two elements, with outcomes left until last, and then usually not assessed well. Now, the focus is outcome based.

Structure

Standards to measure structure focus on what needs to be done in order to provide care. Examples of standards include the number and qualification of staff members, resources, supplies, and productivity.

Process

Process standards describe how the care should be provided, or what nursing actions are used to provide the care. Examples of process elements are staff satisfaction, pain management, maintenance of skin integrity, client education, discharge planning, and responsiveness to unplanned client care needs.

Outcome

Outcome standards identify the desired outcome of nursing care. Examples of outcomes are morbidity/mortality rate, length of stay, adverse incidents, attainment of specific client outcomes, secondary complications, client satisfaction, and client adherence to discharge plan.

Continuity of Care

Continuity of care is to ensure that all appropriate care is provided at the appropriate time. All care flows on a continuum so that one shift adequately and succinctly reports to the oncoming shift in order to provide uninterrupted care. The evaluation of this is an integral part of quality improvement.

Continuous Quality Improvement (CQI)

Quality assurance programs of the past typically focused on problem detection and focused primarily on clinical outcomes and minimum standards. Because this process was chiefly reactionary in nature, the quality improvement movement began in an effort to raise standards of care rather than simply identify when minimum standards have not been met. Thus, continuous quality improvement (CQI) is a process in which ongoing analysis laid the foundation for change and improvement. Continuous quality improvement (CQI) or total quality management (TQM) includes all activities of quality assurance, but moves a step further to include programs aimed at improving quality of care (not just correcting the error) and problem prevention. In this way, the approach is proactive versus reactive, and the focus is on continual improvement. The aim of continuous quality improvement is to evaluate and improve care through the system versus faulting an individual or group. In this way, CQI programs focus on quality by design (prevention), rather than quality by inspection (correction). Throughout the process, it is important to build on the organization's strengths.

Steps in the CQI Monitoring and Evaluation Process:

- Assigning responsibility
- Delineating scope of practice
- Identifying important aspects of care
- Identifying indicators
- Establishing means to trigger evaluation
- Collecting and organizing data
- Initiating evaluation
- Taking action to improve care
- Assessing the effectiveness of the action
- Communicating results
- Identifying breakdowns
- Documenting client care and results of interventions on the appropriate record or flow sheet

Standards and Other Tools

Standards and other tools, such as practice guidelines, evidence-based practice, protocols, and clinical pathways are all useful in establishing criteria and data collection about quality of care. Sources of standards include internal criteria developed by the organization, as well as position descriptions, policies and procedures, goals employees identify during performance appraisals, and other guidelines that are discussed in this section (protocols, clinical pathways). External sources like the standards developed by professional organizations, accreditation organizations, and government regulations are also used to establish guidelines for quality care. External standards must be adjusted to apply to an individual organization. This is particularly important for standards developed by professional organizations.

A standard is an authoritative statement that describes the specific responsibilities, skills, and knowledge possessed by members of a profession. Standards of care are written to reflect the quality level considered adequate for the profession and include the following:

Standards of Practice: The focus is competency of practice for safe delivery of care to the public. The standards of practice are determined by the professional nursing organizations, such as the American Nurses Association (ANA), and reflect the values, priorities, roles, and foundation for professional nursing practice. The ANA Standards of Clinical Nursing Practice is the global framework for the general standards of nursing practice; a means to evaluate practice for ongoing monitoring and quality improvement; and a way for nursing to be accountable to the public. The ANA and other specialty organizations publish standards for the many specialty areas, such as neonatal nursing, oncology nursing, rehabilitation, and school nursing. The specific duties are regulated by the Nurse Practice Act in each state and include detailed descriptions and listings of permissible nursing activities, including general nursing (RN, PN) and advance practice roles (e.g., nurse practitioners, nurse midwife and nurse anesthetists).

Standards of Professional Performance: Formal description of what constitutes competent level of behavior in the professional role, including activities related to quality improvement, performance appraisal, education, ethics, collaboration, research, and resource utilization.

Clinical Practice Guidelines: Statements used to assist nursing professionals to make decisions about the care they provide to persons with various health care problems. As a method to improve the quality of care, professional organizations and the federal government, such as the Agency for Healthcare Research and Quality, have published extensive guidelines to identify outcomes of interventions. Also, the U.S. Department of Health and Human Services (a federal agency) impacts nursing practice by regulating hospitals and long-term care facilities.

Evidenced-Based Practice: Evidence-based practice (EBP) is the use of high-quality, clinically relevant scientific research to improve clinical nursing practice and client care. Research findings are reviewed, analyzed, and summarized for use in the client care setting. These summaries are called "evidence syntheses," "systematic reviews," or "integrative reviews" depending on the organization that prepares the summary. An evidence synthesis integrates research findings into a single conclusion that a nurse, physician, or a medical organization can use to plan client care. Nursing care that is based on scientific evidence is more effective and produces better client outcomes than care that is simply based on tradition, opinions, personal experience, and trial and error. However, nurses still need to combine EBP with their own clinical experience and each client's unique problems to produce a truly effective and realistic plan of care.

Clinical Pathways: Systematic description or schematic representations of specific care decisions for medical or nursing health care issues. They are designed to control health care costs and focus on the measurement of outcomes. More importantly, clinical pathways are important for improving client outcomes by improving morbidity and mortality and other outcomes. This benchmarking method for individual clients was developed to standardize care to better monitor costs and client outcomes. It also determines the sources and degree of variance between the usual and customary care and the care that is actually delivered. Commonalities regarding specific disease or procedures such as ventilator management or coronary artery bypass surgery truly define clinical pathways. The guidelines or pathways identify specific continuity of care such as labs, nursing and ancillary care needed, length of stay, etc. that all clients are expected to receive. The pathway goals and plan are based on evidence-based medicine and nursing, as well as research and regional experiences and resources. The purpose of clinical practice guidelines, evidence-based medicine, and clinical pathways is to provide the best quality of care that is also the most appropriate and affordable.

Benchmarking

Benchmarking is a data-driven type of quality improvement program used to identify areas for increasing the quality and efficiency in the delivery of health care services. A climate for attaining the shared mission and vision of the organization is fostered with the benchmarking approach. This approach utilizes the standards of care and practice protocols, clinical pathways, accreditation standards, and other quality assurance documentation for ensuring optimum level of services. The organization compares performance within the organization to outcomes and cost containment and identifies key areas for improvement. In the competitive market today, this type of performance-based approach can also be used to compare ideas and services to external organizations. Benchmarking is one way to identify the opportunities to meet the demand for better-quality products and services.

Benchmarking also involves the development of critical (clinical) pathways. Critical pathways are systematic descriptions or schematic representations of specific care decisions for medical or nursing health care issues. They are designed to control health care costs and focus on the measurement of outcomes. This benchmarking method for individual clients was developed to standardize the care to better monitor costs. It also determines the sources and degree of variance between the usual and customary care, and the care that is actually delivered.

Utilization Review

Utilization review (UR) is the process of assessing medical necessity, appropriateness of health care services in a particular setting, and efficiency of care. UR focus includes the reason for admission to a facility, type and extent of treatment, length of hospitalization, and discharge planning and follow-up considerations.

Culturally and Linguistically Appropriate Services (CLAS)

The national standards for Culturally and Linguistically Appropriate Services (CLAS) were developed by the U.S. Department of Health and Human Services and the Office of Minority Health. These standards were first published in the Federal Register in December 2000. The purpose of the national CLAS standards is to correct the inequities that adversely affect the health care traditionally provided to people of color and to members of ethnic groups. The CLAS standards were based on an analytical review of the regulations, contracts, laws, and standards that affected the health care of minorities in the United States. The goal of the CLAS standards is to provide better health care to all individuals and to eliminate discrimination against minorities by health care providers and health care organizations.

Groups that use CLAS standards include:
- Nurses and other health care providers
- Professional organizations such as the American Nurses Association, the American Medical Association, and the National Association of Social Work
- Accrediting agencies such as the Joint Commission on Accreditation of Healthcare Organizations (JCAHO) and the National Committee on Quality Assurance (NCQA)
- Policy makers on the local, state and federal levels
- Educators in human service professions such as nursing, medicine, law and social work
- Client advocates

Accreditation

Accreditation is the standardized program for the evaluation of health care organizations. It is based on the established minimum standards for quality health care. The accreditation process is voluntary; however, the distinction offers benefits to the provider. For example, hospitals that have achieved various levels of accreditation may serve the community as a teaching facility for nursing and medical students. Fiscal ramifications are directly related to obtaining accreditation status. The public perception of a health care institution is related to the seal of quality awarded by the accrediting body. The Joint Commission on Accreditation of Healthcare Organizations (JCAHO) is the most widely used accreditation body for hospitals.

Magnet Status

The Magnet Recognition Program for Nursing Excellence is a program administered through the American Nurses Credentialing Center and combines quality indicators identified by the American Nurses Association and the Scope and Standards for Nurse Administrators to both quantitatively and qualitatively measure nursing services in a health care organization. Magnet status, with its link between quality client care and nursing excellence, is now viewed as the single most effective mechanism for providing customers and nurses with comparative information. It is considered a seal of approval for quality nursing care. Nurses in hospitals that have been awarded magnet status generally exhibit greater levels of autonomy, more control over the practice setting, and better relationships with the health care team, especially physicians.

Staff Education

Credentialing and competency are important factors when considering staff education and staff selection. **Credentialing** refers to licensure, certification, and academic degrees related to the job. It is important to recognize that none of these credentialing methods ensure ongoing competency. **Competency** is the demonstration of knowledge and skills in meeting professional role expectations and outcomes for care. In a hospital setting, nurses are usually evaluated on some competencies on an annual basis, or more often depending on the skill.

To ensure safe delivery of care to the public and improve the quality of health care services, nursing professionals must continually update clinical skills and knowledge. The nurse must commit to a lifelong learning style. There are several approaches to staff education:

In-service education: Instruction or training to assist the nurse in performing necessary skills in the work setting as well as updating the nurse on infection control, fire and safety, and confidentiality issues. Examples of educational programs include:

- Orientation
- Demonstration of new equipment, supplies or procedures
- Practice of previously learned skills and safety procedures
- Provision of programmed instruction booklets that includes a post-test for nurses to complete and return

Continuing education: Planned, organized learning experiences designed to increase the knowledge and skills for competency-based practice. Methods of delivery for continuing education may include the traditional group classroom setting, Internet-based, conference, or self-study program. Many states require documentation of continuing education to maintain licensure; professional certifying bodies for specialized areas of practice also mandate continuing education for certification.

Academic education: Formal education occurring within the higher education setting (e.g., college or university), preceptorships

What should you look for when you are deciding to attend or participate in a continuing education program?

Accreditation of the program: Who is providing the continuing education credits?

Faculty biography: Qualifications regarding expertise in the content area

Content, course objectives: Reasonableness of time to deliver content, and program format (e.g., workshop, panel, self-study, distance learning via internet, etc.)

Cost: Who pays for the course, and whether reimbursement will be made for tuition, transportation, and time spent at the conference

Convenience: Location and time

Relevance and interest in clinical practice area

Management and the Learning Environment

An important managerial function involves the provision of staff development through educational programs and mentorship opportunities. For effective learning and instruction, concepts of adult learning are critical. The learning needs of the adult are unique; many adults have benefited from experience, development of critical thinking skills related to real life problems, maturity and self-directed goals, and internal motivation. The nurse manager who incorporates these traits into the learning environment is likely to be more successful. An attitude of inquiry and flexibility to customize the instruction to the learner's needs promotes habits of lifelong learning.

Mentorship for Adult Learning

Mentorship is an effective method of fostering the development and professional career of an individual. Nurse mentors are experienced, competent professionals who develop a genuine relationship to provide information, support, advice, and exemplary learning to a novice nurse. This relationship is characterized primarily by commitment to growth and development. The mentor helps the novice to attain professional goals by:

- Broadening the novice's viewpoint
- Increasing understanding of a topic, situation, or problem
- Helping the novice to sharpen critical thinking skills
- Examining ideas and analyzing problems thoroughly
- Aiding in the formulation of a sound plan of action
- Stimulating the novice to make informed decisions
- Building confidence and a sense of self-efficacy
- Giving honest feedback, including evaluation about day-to-day encounters
- Networking with others in positions of power or decision-making
- Providing new opportunities for growth in professional practice

Critical Thinking Exercise: Quality Improvement

1. Compare and contrast organizational structure, process, and outcomes as they apply to quality.

2. What is a clinical pathway?

3. If you work in the Utilization Review department, what types of data might you collect?

4. What is your opinion of health care accreditation?

5. Give an example of applying research findings in nurse practice (evidence-based practice).

CHAPTER 12

Ethical Issues

Key Points

- Ethical issues are common in health care delivery, and nurses confront them daily.
- The goal in ethical reasoning is to reach a mutual, peaceful agreement, that is in the best interests of the client.
- Moral frameworks or theories are consequence-based, principles-based, and relationship-based.
- Moral principles focus on autonomy, nonmaleficence, beneficence, justice, fidelity, and veracity.
- Values influence both clients' and nurses' decisions.
- The American Nurses Association's *Code for Nurses with Interpretive Statements* is used as a guideline for nurses as they confront ethical issues.
- Ethics committees are used by many health care organizations to assist staff with ethical dilemmas.

Overview

In their day-to-day work, nurses often encounter ethical problems/situations in which the question is not, "What should be done?" but, "Should I do this?" Moral problems are created as a result of technological advances, societal changes, and nurses' conflicting obligations to clients, families, employers, primary care providers, and other nurses. Sometimes an ethical problem exists because the nurse is not sure what is "right." In other instances, the nurse may feel sure of the right action, but cannot carry out that action without great personal risk (e.g., losing her/his job).

When moral problems arise, the nurse's input is important. However, many people are usually involved in making an ethical decision. Therefore, collaboration, communication, and compromise are important skills. The goal of ethical reasoning in nursing is to reach a beneficial agreement that is in the best interest of the client. Nurses must maintain a nonjudgmental attitude, be honest, respect and support client decisions, and protect the privacy and confidentiality of the client.

Morality: Usually refers to private, personal standards of what is right and wrong. Moral issues involve important social values and norms, not trivial things. They can be recognized by an aroused conscience and/or feelings, such as guilt, hope, or shame; or the tendency to respond to the situation with performance words like ought, should, right, wrong, good, and bad. Morality and ethics are often used interchangeably, although philosophers and ethicists distinguish between them.

> **Ethics**: Refers to a method of inquiry about the rightness/wrongness of human actions, the practices or beliefs of a group, and the standards of moral behavior described in the group's formal code of ethics.
>
> **Bioethics**: Ethics as applied to "life situations" (e.g., decisions about euthanasia, prolonging life, abortion).
>
> **Nursing ethics**: Ethical issues that occur in the context of nursing practice questions that nurses must address with regard to their own actions.
>
> **Values**: Freely chosen, long-lasting beliefs or attitudes about the worth of something (e.g., a person or an idea).
>
> **Value system**: A personal set of beliefs on a continuum from most to least important that form the value system, give it direction, and provides the basis for decisions and choices.

Moral Frameworks (Theories)

Nurses use moral theories to guide their ethical decision-making. Moral theories can be differentiated by their emphasis on either consequences of an action, principles, and duties, or relationships.

Consequence-based (teleological) theories judge the "rightness" of an action based on the consequences it produces.

Utilitarianism (a consequentialist theory) views a good act as one that brings the least harm and the most good to the most people.

Principle-based (deontological) theories emphasize individual rights, duties, and obligations. They judge an action independently of its results. An action is moral if it follows an impartial, objective principle.

Relationship-based (caring) theories stress courage, generosity, commitment, and the need to nurture and maintain relationships. Caring theories promote the common good or the welfare of the group, rather than stressing individual rights.

A moral framework guides moral decisions, but does not determine the outcome of a decision. Two nurses using the same framework might make entirely different decisions about a situation.

Moral Principles

Moral principles are statements about broad concepts such as autonomy and justice. Even though people disagree about the right action to take, they may be able to agree on the principles that apply—this can be the basis for discussion and an acceptable compromise. For example, most people would agree on the principle that nurses should tell the truth to clients (veracity), even if they disagree as to whether the nurse should deceive a particular client about his or her prognosis. However, in some institutions or parts of the country, questions regarding the client's medical care (e.g., results of diagnostics or life and death issues such as cancer) may not be questions that the nurse has the "authority" to answer. Some basic principles are:

Autonomy: The right to make one's own decisions; the right to choose personal goals. This means that nurses respect a client's right to make decisions, even when those choices seem not to be in the client's best interest. It also means treating clients with consideration and respect. In the health care setting, informed consent is a direct application of the ethical principle. The client who declines treatment or discharges against medical advice (AMA) exercises autonomous rights.

Nonmaleficence: The duty to do no harm. Harm includes "risk of harm," which is not always clear. For example, a nursing intervention that is meant to be helpful may have a harmful side effect.

Beneficence: "Doing good." Nurses are obligated to implement actions that benefit clients and families.

Justice: Fairness. Nurses often face decisions that call for a sense of fairness. They must weigh the facts carefully to divide their time fairly among the clients they care for during a workday.

Fidelity: Keeping promises and agreements.

Veracity: Telling the truth. Honesty in disclosure is essential at all levels of professional practice.

Respect for others: Includes the client's right for self-determination. Sensitivity to cultural, religious, and lifestyle diversity transcends respectful nursing practice.

Although principles are important, they may conflict sometimes. For example, telling the truth (veracity) to a client may cause the client to become anxious and hypertensive (violating the principle of nonmaleficence).

Values

Values are an integral part of ethical decision-making. The formation of a person's values is influenced by external factors, such as environment, time, education, and resources. Cultural, religious, and generational sources also play an important part in shaping a person's professional, organizational, and personal values. Values (conscious or unconscious) underlie all moral decisions.

Ethical principles that are essential to professional practice include:

Altruism: The desire or act of doing good for another, including commitment and caring

Equality: Sameness of state or continued course, uniformity, evenness

Justice: The ethical principle that persons who have similar circumstances and conditions should be treated alike

Truth: Faithfulness to fact or reality; relating to accountability, honesty and rationality

Human dignity: The intrinsic worthiness of human beings, irrespective of age, sex, physical or mental ability, religion, ethnic or social origin

Human rights: Self-determination, privacy, freedom

Aesthetics: Appreciation, creativity, sensitivity, imagination

Freedom: Capacity to exercise choice

Altruism: Unselfish regard or concern for the welfare of another person

Method for Professional Decision-Making

Ethical decision-making is a process that commonly involves following steps that closely resemble the nursing process:

- Clearly identify the problem.
- Consider the causative factors, additive variable, precipitating events, and possible implications of the problem.
- Explore various options for action.
- Select the most appropriate plan for dealing with the ethical dilemma.
- Implement the decided course of action while maintaining sensitivity to the complexities of the problem.
- Evaluate the results or consequences of interventions/decisions.

Common Ethical Issues Involving Nurses

The ANA Center for Ethics and Human Rights and other authorities have identified the following as some of the ethical problems that nurses encounter most frequently:

- Cost-containment issues that jeopardize client welfare and access to health care (allocation of scarce resources)
- End-of-life decisions
- Breaches of client confidentiality (e.g., computerized information management)
- Use of advance directives, informed consent, and procedures
- Issues in the care of HIV/AIDS clients
- Abortion and selective termination
- Organ transplantation
- Rationing of care
- Reproductive therapies
- Providing medical information to the client
- Enactment of the HIPAA policies
- End-of-life pain control issues (e.g., full and effective doses of pain medication should not be withheld from clients at the end of life, even if giving them might hasten death)

Ethical Responsibilities of the Manager

A manager's functions and responsibilities materialize from a complex set of interactions among self, the organization, the community, and society. Therefore, it is not surprising that nursing management in health care today involves many ethical components. Increasing autonomy, advocacy roles, and professional accountability will continue to add complexity to ethical dilemmas that nurse managers must face now and in the future. The primary ethical dilemma facing most nurse managers is balancing the responsibility of ensuring the delivery of safe, high-quality care with the fiscal responsibilities of their administrative roles.

Because scientific advances and limited resources create new complexities and ethical dilemmas, nurse managers must act as the client advocate with regard to the distribution of resources. The manager also has a responsibility to assist staff in dealing with ethical issues to create a climate in the work environment where ethical behavior is the minimum standard. The nurse manager must be able to ask the right questions and risk doing the right thing in every phase of the management process. The effective manager recognizes the importance of using ethical principles for decision-making in the practice setting.

Nursing Codes of Ethics and Standards of Professional Performance

A code of ethics is a formal statement of the ethical values and principles that are shared by members of a group. It provides a standard for professional actions. *Nursing Codes of Ethics*, including the *International Council of Nurses' Code for Nurses* and the *ANA Code for Nurses with Interpretative Statements*, give guidance in terms of ethical accountability for nurse's actions within the scope of professional practice. The present code reflects a commitment to the principles of respect for autonomy, beneficence, nonmaleficence, justice, veracity, fidelity, and confidentiality. Codes of ethics are not legally enforceable, and they are only as effective as the nurses who use them. They are general, so even though they provide guidance for ethical decision-making, codes of ethics do not guarantee the "right" answer in any given situation. However, they may be referred to in courts of law.

Ethics Committees

Many institutions have ethics committees that provide education, policy making, case review, and consultation. Usually they are multidisciplinary and thus create a forum for widely differing views. Nurses' input into these committees is important, since they often have the most intimate knowledge of the client and situation. For example, staff nurses in a neurology intensive care unit are concerned and raise several questions about the moral issue of taking clients off ventilators and declaring them "brain dead." The nurses in these cases should contact the hospital ethics committee.

In some health care organizations, such as home health care agencies, hospices, and sub- acute centers, many executives employ the services of an ombudsman. This person is usually a community leader, such as a minister, who serves as an outside party to offer advice and counsel on ethical issues for the organization.

Critical Thinking Exercise: Ethical Issues

Situation: You are caring for M. J., who has terminal lung cancer and is receiving hospice care. He is 45 years old, married, and has two children, ages 5 and 7. He has smoked since he was 17 and continues to smoke. His father died of lung cancer. His wife tells you that M. J. has always been concerned about his appearance. Due to chemotherapy, he has lost weight as well as his hair.

1. Based on these facts and on what you know about cancer, discuss how moral principles and values might affect your care of M.J.

Situation: Mrs. P. has a history of osteoporosis. She fell in her home, sustaining a compound fracture of her left hip. She was admitted to the hospital for surgical hip repair. Her husband is extremely anxious about his wife's condition. On returning Mrs. P. from the recovery room, the transport attendant inadvertently left the chart in her room. Later, the RN found Mr. P. seated at his wife's bedside, reading the chart.

2. What ethical principle was violated?

3. How would you manage this situation as the RN caring for Mrs. P.?

CHAPTER 13

Legal Issues

Key Points

- Nurses are legally responsible and accountable for assessing, diagnosing, planning, implementing, and evaluating nursing care.
- Nurses need to understand legal issues related to health care and to adhere to legal guidelines.
- Sources of law are the U.S. Constitution, state constitutions, state and federal legislation (laws, statutes, regulations), and common law.
- The types of law are public and private. Criminal law is a form of public law. Private law is also known as civil law and includes both unintentional and intentional damages.
- Risk management is used to limit an organization's legal risk.
- The doctrine of respondent superior establishes the employer as responsible for the employee's actions.
- State boards of nursing establish nurse practice acts to regulate the scope of nursing practice.

Overview

Understanding of nursing law is important to ensure that the nurse's actions are in compliance with established standards of care; adherence to these guidelines will serve to protect the nurse from liability. To avoid professional liability, the nurse must provide services within the legally defined scope of practice. A highly effective strategy to prevent a potential lawsuit is fostering good communication and trust in the nurse-client relationship. The satisfied client is less likely to pursue legal discourse than the disgruntled client. Nurses may be involved in a medical malpractice case by testifying as a defendant on behalf of his/her own actions in direct client care or as a witness for actions/decisions of another member of the health care team. The nurse may serve as an expert witness by providing testimony to the judge and jury regarding the standards for nursing care and the nature of usual and customary action.

Law Basics

Functions of the Law in Nursing

- Accountability helps to maintain a minimum standard of nursing practice.
- Differentiates nurses' responsibilities from those of other health care professionals
- Specifies which nursing actions are legal in caring for clients

Sources of Law

The U.S. Constitution is the supreme law of the United States. It contains legal rights and responsibilities, and is the foundation for the judicial system. Each state constitution is a major source of law for the state.

Legislation (statutes) consists of laws enacted by federal, state, or other legislative bodies or agencies (e.g., the U. S. Senate, state legislature, agencies such as Health Care Financing Administration and the Food and Drug Administration). When federal and state laws conflict, federal law prevails. State law regulates nursing practices within a state through nurse practice acts.

Common (case) law is law that evolves from court decisions. This system of jurisprudence is based on precedents set in previous, similar cases. Common law is often used to resolve disputes between two parties, based on principles of justice, reason, and common good.

Types of Law

Public law is a body of law that deals with relationships between individuals and the government.

Criminal law is a type of public law that deals with the safety and welfare of the public (e.g., homicide, rape, and theft) and has imprisonment as a possible consequence.

Private (civil) law is the body of law that deals with relationships between private persons.

Contract law enforces agreements, while tort law defines duties and rights among individuals that are not based on contracts. Examples of tort law relevant to nurses are negligence, malpractice, invasion of privacy, and assault and battery.

Statutory law involves legislature established by federal, state or local governing bodies that regulate employment issues such as health and retirement benefits, and workers' compensation.

Civil Law in Health Care Delivery

Unintentional Torts

- Liability refers to the responsibility for acts of commission and omission.
- Negligence is the failure to provide the care that an ordinary, reasonable, and prudent person would perform under similar circumstances, which places another person at risk for harm.
- Gross negligence involves an extreme breach of care, in which the practitioner clearly places another at risk for injury.
- Malpractice is negligent action that occurs while a person is performing in the professional role. In order for malpractice to be proven, the following four elements must be present:
  - The nurse has a relationship with the client that involves providing care (e.g., has been assigned to care for the client in the hospital).
  - The nurse failed to observe a standard of care in the specific situation.
  - The client sustained harm, injury, or damage.

- The harm must have occurred as a direct result of the nurse's failure to act in accordance with a prevalent professional standard of care. The nurse with the necessary expertise and skills should foresee the potential harm of the action.

Intentional Torts

Assault is an attempt or threat to touch another person without justification (e.g., a nurse threatens, "If you don't eat, we'll have to force feed you.").

Battery is the intentional physical contact with a person or object the person is holding or wearing. To qualify as battery, the touching must be wrongful in some way, such as embarrassing, causing injury, or done without permission (e.g., continuing to bathe a client after the client has said, "Stop").

Informed consent implies that:

- Consent was voluntary and free of coercion.
- The client was competent and of legal age.
- The client had enough information for an appraisal of the nature, risks, benefits, potential application, procedure, and potential complications of the procedure to make an informed choice.

Failure to obtain an informed consent may result in an intentional tort.

False imprisonment is restraining or detaining another person against his or her will. For example, a nurse cannot detain a client who insists upon leaving the hospital against medical advice. The client has a right to leave even though it may be harmful to him or her. This does not apply if the client is incompetent or committed, which requires a legal process. Instead of false imprisonment, then, it is a matter of protecting the client from injury.

Areas of Potential Liability

Nurses should seek legal counsel from the health care organization's risk management or a personal attorney when experiencing legal issues.

Invasion of privacy: Nurses may be liable if they breach confidentiality or intrude into a client's private domain (e.g., by taking photographs without permission). Confidentially refers to the privacy of information and its ethical use. As a result of the Health Insurance Portability and Accountability Act (HIPAA) of 1996, federal privacy standards are now in place to make sure that healthcare providers protect the privacy and security of client's health information, personla data, and medical records. Clients must be informed of their health care provider's privacy practices, and all employees of the provider must adhere to established standards for safeguarding client's confidentiality and privacy at all times. Access to this information must be limited to only those individuals or organizations that require some or all of the information for certain identified purposes, such as treatment or billing.

Loss of client property

Unprofessional conduct (e.g., falsification of client records, illegal use of controlled substances)

Good Samaritan Acts: Laws designed to protect health care workers who give assistance in an emergency. In the U.S., most state laws do not require a person to give aid to someone in distress—it is considered more of a moral, rather than a legal, duty. Most states do have legislation protecting a "Good Samaritan" from legal liability for injuries caused under these circumstances. Nurses who choose to render emergency care should:

- Limit actions to first aid, if possible.
- Not perform actions with which they are unfamiliar.
- Offer help, but do not insist.
- Stay at the scene until the injured party leaves or until relieved by another qualified person.

Scope of Practice: Refers to the legally permissible boundaries of practice, as defined by the state practice act or other legal statutes.

Job Abandonment: Not following health care organization policy regarding staffing and responsibility of covering client care.

Refusal to "float": Reluctance to provide care when and if you, the nurse, feels unqualified to provide such care. The nurse must communicate to the manager or supervisor and follow organization policy. Continued problems may be reported to the state board of nursing or union, if unionized.

Notifying primary care provider: Whenever the nurse notifies the primary care provider, he/she must document the reason for which contact was made, date, time, and result. If it is an emergency or the primary care provider is needed for decision- making and the primary care provider cannot be reached, this must be communicated to the supervisor and the occurrence documented.

Patient Self-Determination Act: Law requiring that all individuals who receive medical care in a health care facility recognized by Medicare and Medicaid must be provided with written information about their legal right to make health care decisions, including accepting or refusing medical or surgical treatment. It is the nurse's legal and ethical responsibility to provide clients with information about their right to formulate advance directives, and other legal documents that effect their medical and nursing care.

Advance Directives: Legal documents that contain written instructions concerning the type and extent of future medical care the client wants to receive. Advance directives should be monitored by the physician and hospital staff. Many hospitals now request advance directives from the client upon admission. If the client has not prepared advance directives, a basic explanation should be provided by the nurse. The nurse should ask the client if he/she would like to speak with a specially designated staff member who can explain all of the legal issues. Inform the client that this person will help to draw up the advance directives and notarize the documents. Note the client's decision in regard to advance directives in the client's record. Major types of advance directives include:

- **Living wills**: Living wills are documents instructing health care providers to withhold or withdraw life-sustaining procedures when death is imminent. Living wills may also list procedures the person wants done when death is imminent. Each state has its own requirements for living wills. Generally, two witnesses (not necessarily relatives or health care providers) are needed when the client signs the document.

- **Durable power of attorney**: Durable power of attorney for health care is a legal document that lists the person or persons designated by a client to make health decisions when the client is no longer able to make informed decisions because of an incapacitating medical condition. This document allows the person with power of attorney to make bank transactions, sign Social Security checks, apply for disability, and write checks for the client who is ill.
- **Health care proxy**: This is a legal document that is used in some states instead of a durable power of attorney for health care.
- **Do Not Attempt to Resuscitate Order (DNAR):** This order may be written by a physician, usually in consultation with the client's family or significant others. A DNAR order directs the staff not to attempt to resuscitate a client in the event of sudden cardiopulmonary arrest. In some states and institutions, the physician may write a DNAR order when the client does not have a living will. It is important for the nurse to be aware of state and institutional requirements concerning DNAR orders because they vary.

Child and elder abuse reporting: Mandated federal law requires that suspected child and elder abuse must be reported to appropriate state authorities.

Ownership of medical records: Medical records are the property of the health care organization; however, the client has a right to view those records and must give consent in order for information to be shared with others outside the organization, unless ordered by court to share the information. There are recent new regulations about client consent, and this area requires that health care professionals update their current knowledge about consent.

Confidentiality: Refers to the privacy of information and the ethical use of client information. With the exception of client threats of harm to self or others, clients can expect confidentiality. Information about clients or information from their medical records may not be shared with anyone who is not directly involved in their care. The right of confidentiality includes protection of the client's privacy. Based on the Health Insurance Portability and Accountability Act (HIPAA) of 1996, clients have the right to request that an organization does not confirm that a client is present or is being treated at a facility.

Chemical dependency in staff: Controlled medication is monitored according to state regulations. Health care organizations and professionals must follow these regulations. Health care professionals who are abusing substances must be reported to supervisory staff.

Sexual harassment: An increasing problem. Federal laws protect persons from sexual harassment.

Delegation: Involves empowering others to perform a task for the shared goal of the group. There is a risk of liability with delegation, which involves the skills and experience of the individual to which the task is delegated. It also depends on the type of task delegated, regulations and practice acts, and policies and procedures. Appropriate selection and monitoring of the delegate's performance is essential to avoid liability.

Refusal to treat: When a health care organization/professional refuses to treat a client, the client must not be at risk for death or permanent injury. The client must be stabilized before transfer or referral. When a "refusal to treat" is enforced, it should be documented. Federal laws dictate what must occur in these circumstances.

Documentation: The medical record is a legal document. Nurses are responsible for maintaining accurate and complete records of care provided and client responses to care. Falsification of records is illegal, including omission of relevant information. An example of an error of commission would be intentionally documenting fictitious vital signs when vital signs had not been taken. If corrections are made, do not destroy what was written. The original documentation should still be legible and clearly marked to indicate any changes that have been made with date, time, and person identified.

Primary care provider orders: Nurses are expected to ask for clarification of ambiguous or seemingly erroneous orders. Otherwise, they are expected to carry out the order exactly as written.

Age discrimination: Federal law prohibits discrimination against persons over age 40 unless reasonable factors affecting performance as related to job performance are present.

Incident/irregular occurrence reports: An incident is any event that does not conform to the routine operation of a health care unit or the routine care of a client. Variances typically involve potential or actual harm -- either to the client, a visitor, or an employee, and some degree of risk to the institution. Common occurrences that require incidence reports are client falls, accidental needle-stick injuries, illness or injury of visitors, employee injuries, medication administration errors, accidental omission of ordered therapies, and carelessness during a procedure that led to injury or risk for the client. An incident report must be prepared when an incidence occurs, even when no one appears to be injured. An incidence report documents situations for which the institution is potentially liable. Most institutions have a specific incident report form for this purpose. The healthcare provider who witnessed the incident should complete the report in full detail as soon as possible after the incident. If a person is injured, the nurse must first ensure the person's safety. A physician will then examine the person to determine if any injury has occurred. The incident report should contain only objective data. When possible, the nurse should report the client's view of what happened, using the client's own words. The report should also contain the nurse's observation of the situation. Like all legal documents, the report should be legible and factual and should be worded so that no one is blamed for the incident. Incidence reports are kept on file to identify when incidents occur, the sequence of events, client response, actions taken, and the results. Incident reports can be requested for review in malpractice cases.

Variance reports: A variance is any event that does not conform to the routine operation of a health care unit or to the routine care of a client. Variances typically involve potential or actual harm — either to the client, a visitor, or an employee, and some degree of risk to the institution. A variance report must be prepared when an incidence occurs, even when no one appears to be injured. Most institutions have a specific report form for this purpose. The healthcare provider who witnessed the event should complete the report in full detail as soon as possible after it occurs.

Medication errors: Health care organizations require that staff members who identify a medication error complete an incident report. Completion of this report should not be documented in the medical record. Objective reporting of the sequence of events and client's health status are documented. (e.g., Client did not receive 9 a.m. dose of Digoxin. Primary care provider informed. Digoxin given at 1 p.m., as ordered).

Risk management: Many health care organizations have risk management departments. Major functions of the risk management department include:

- Identifying situations that place the agency at financial risk or may result in a lawsuit.
- Investigating and analyzing problems and incidents.
- Determining the type and frequency of incidents.
- Minimizing losses after a client care error is documented. Financial losses may occur as a result of malpractice or the cost of an extended length of stay for the client. Additional losses include negative public opinion and employee dissatisfaction.
- Identifying opportunities to improve client care
- Participating on hospital committees, such as the Patient Safety Committee, Pharmacy and Nursing Committee, Ethics Committee, and other agency committees that develop programs to reduce risks. Each nurse is also a risk manager. By minimizing risks when providing care for clients, the nurse reduces the possibility that clients will be financially and emotionally devastated by poor care. The nurse also helps the institution avoid lawsuits by ensuring a safe environment for care. When a incidence does occur, the nurse should immediately notify the risk management department and prepare an incidence report form as mandated by institutional policies and procedures. Employee complaints of harassment or discrimination should also be promptly reported to supervisors and the risk management department. Such complaints can expose the institution to bad publicity and the possibility of lawsuits.

Client rights: Client rights is an ever-evolving area of nursing and medical practice that is becoming increasingly standardized and regulated by the federal government as well as by accrediting agencies that define client rights. Many organizations have prepared statements that list client rights. In addition, each health care agency must display in a public area the American Hospital Association's document entitled "A Patient's Bill of Rights." Clients have the right to:

- Access to health care when needed
- Considerate, respectful and nondiscriminatory care
- Receive emergency care in an emergency department of a hospital, regardless of whether that hospital is designated as one of the insurance carrier's preferred providers
- Receive accurate and easily understood information

- An interpreter if the client does not speak English
- Perform culture-specific practices as long as the practice does not harm the client or others
- Assistance if the client has difficulty communicating, or has a physical or mental disability
- Be informed of all treatment options
- Participate in decisions about their care
- Choose a parent, guardian, family member or other individual as a representative if the client cannot make informed decisions
- Review their medical records and receive a copy. If a client believes a medical record is not accurate, the client can request that the record be amended.
- Expect an objective review of any complaint against physicians, hospitals, or health care staff. This includes complaints about waiting times, operating hours, staff conduct, and the adequacy of the facility.
- Refuse care. Based on the ethical principle of autonomy, any client who is competent may refuse care.

Informed consent: A potential area for liability, informed consent is voluntary permission from the client with regard to a procedure or surgery. The primary care provider is responsible for informing the client about the procedure, its potential benefits and risks, and obtaining the client's consent. Two criteria must be satisfied for informed consent:

- The person(s) giving consent must fully understand the procedure, risks, expected outcomes, possible side effects, and alternative treatments.
- An individual who is considered legally capable must give consent. (e.g., competent adult, legal guardian, emancipated minor, parent, court order).

Technology advances: These afford much potential for liability. **Fax machines** should be in an area away from the public. As a general rule, when confidential or sensitive information is faxed, it should be preceded by a telephone call to the receiving area to ensure that an employee retrieves it and places it in the appropriate medical record. **E-mail communications** must be handled with discretion. Care should be taken with regard to messages put into electronic format. (Novice personnel have been known to hit the "send all" button, only to discover that the message has been sent to all hospital departments.)

Organ donation: People who are legally competent can decide if they want to donate their bodies or organs for medical purposes after they die. There are legal documents that individuals can sign if they wish to donate their organs. In many states, adults can sign the back of their driver's license to indicate their intention to donate. However, in other states, the client's family will need to give consent for organ donation after the person's death, or they can revoke the deceased person's consent to donate. Most states have request laws. Request laws stipulate that at the time of a person's death, a designated health care provider, called a trained requestor, must ask family members to consider organ or tissue donation.

Required request laws were enacted because there was a shortage of organs for transplantation.

When caring for a client whose death is imminent, the nurse should first check the client's record for any documents that address organ donation. If there are no documents, then the nurse should contact a specially trained staff member who may legally request organ donation. The nurse should follow the health care agency's policy on when and whom to notify about the brain death or expiration. In addition, the nurse should support the family and client during this difficult time of loss and provide information about organ donation.

State laws determine if a nurse may serve as a witness to the signing of organ donation consent documents. Thus, nurses need to be aware of the organ donation policies and procedures of the institutions where they work, and the laws of the state in which they practice.

Other laws that govern organ donation include the National Organ Transplant Act of 1984 that prohibits the purchase or sale of organs. The Uniform Anatomical Gift Act addresses other issues involved in the removal or transplantation of the client's organs.

Hospitals generally act as donees of anatomical gifts. To coordinate the procurement of anatomical gifts, hospitals are required to establish a agreements with other hospitals and procurement organizations.

Regulation of Nursing Practice

Nursing practice is regulated at the state level, primarily through licensing and nurse practice acts.

Licensure: Legal permit granted by the state boards of nursing in the state of desired employment. Licensure permits an individual demonstrating defined knowledge and skills to practice within a defined scope of practice. In the U.S., licensure is mandatory for employment. It can be revoked for just cause, such as felony or defensible incompetence. The employer and possibly the State Board of Nursing should be notified when concern arises regarding issues related to client safety, substance abuse, and/or health care fraud.

Nurse Practice Acts: Protect the nurse's professional "territory" and legally control nursing practice through licensing. Nurse practice acts define and describe the scope of nursing practice, which protects the public as well as nurses. Each state in the U.S. has a nurse practice act, although they do differ, all require the nurse to be licensed in order to practice.

Accreditation: Process by which the state board of nursing or other private organization (e.g., the National League for Nursing (NLN)) evaluates and approves educational programs or services that meet predetermined criteria. The state boards of nursing must accredit the schools of nursing in the U.S. Most also seek private accreditation (e.g., by the NLN). Accreditation of health care organizations and managed care organizations is very important.

Critical Thinking Exercise: Legal Issues

1. Describe the elements of malpractice and cite an example by applying it to the elements.

2. When would false imprisonment apply to a medical situation?

3. A client was scheduled for surgical removal of one of her ovaries. During the surgery, the surgeon decides the client has a problem with her uterus and removes it. The client's consent for surgery did not mention the uterus. What type of tort is the surgeon liable for under these circumstances?

4. Find out if your state has a Good Samaritan law. If so, what does it cover?

5. You make a medication error by giving the wrong medication to a client. What must you complete after recognizing your error?

6. Should you note in the medical record the completion of this form?

7. What is the difference between an error of omission and an error of commission?

Critical Thinking Exercise Answer Keys

1. Identify the type of leadership power that is used in the following situations.

   a. M.T. is considered to be the unit's source of any information on diabetes. You go to her to ask for help about a newly admitted client with complicated diabetes.

      Expert power: This type of power comes from the respect of individuals' experience and their knowledge, skills and abilities to do a variety of tasks.

   b. The nurse manager in labor and delivery is viewed as the "dictator" by her staff and is known throughout the hospital as someone who is very controlling and restrictive.

      Coercive power: This type of power is used by people in authoritative positions to get what they want at the expense of others, usually subordinates. The power is gained through establishment of fear.

   c. R.B. was hired for the position of nurse manager for a home health agency.

      Legitimate power: This type of power is granted to individuals by the nature of their position within the organization and the duties they are responsible for.

2. M.S. has just taken a new position. She will supervise all of the medical units (four total). Each unit has a nurse manager. What level of management is M.S.'s new position?

   Middle level

Situation: You are applying for a nurse manager position for a neonatal unit in a large academic medical center.

---

3. The position description details the scope of practice for the Nurse Manager position. What would you expect to be the scope of practice for the management position and what management functions would you expect to be listed in order for you to accomplish what the nurse manager position entails?

   The scope of practice for the management position includes supporting and working toward the attainment of the organization's goals and compliance with standards of care and ensuring that employees do the same. The nurse manager organizes, coordinates, and controls staff, fiscal, and other resources. Functions such as leadership, planning, organizing, directing, controlling, recognition, development, advocacy, coordination, staffing, reporting, and budgeting.

4. What skills and competencies would you want to emphasize during your interview?

> **Your critical thinking, communication, and networking skills; managing resources; enhancing employee performance; team-building; evaluating; delegating; clinical and organizational expertise; flexibility; collaboration; and coordination.**

5. You know that you will encounter conflict in your new position. How would you cope with conflict? Would you use any of the coping methods mentioned in this module? Knowing how you have managed conflict in the past, decide how you might handle the following situation: The census for your unit has been low, prompting the need for your nurses to float to other units. You overhear some of your nurses complaining about floating and how they are not enjoying work anymore.

> **This is a personal observation question. There is no correct answer; however, you should think about what you have learned in the module as you re-read your response.**

6. Explain the concept of followership.

> **Followership is an active process that leads to meeting organizational and clinical outcomes. The nurse or nurse manager acquiesce certain tasks such as planning and direction setting to individuals with the specific skill set needed to complete the assignment.**

7. The nurse manager will be implementing a new form of electronic charting. Two nurses, the evening charge nurse and a staff RN are highly skilled in the field of computer technology. They have attended classes at the nearby university on topics related to health services and technology. The nurse manager delegates the task of orienting all nursing staff and troubleshooting the new electronic charting procedure to these two RNs. They are given time to complete the task and the part-time nurses will pick up hours of work to facilitate task accomplishment of the RNs' new duties.

Has the nurse manager delegated the task appropriately?

> **Yes. Since it would probably take a minimum of several weeks to learn about the new charting system and devise an orientation program, the nurse manager found two experts who are already highly skilled at implementing computer technology, and in this case, appropriately delegated the task.client**

What strategies is the nurse manager employing to facilitate this project?

> **Task accomplishment**
> **Team building**
> **Skill recognition of other team members**
> **Meeting organizational goals**

1. You are working on a committee for your home health agency. The purpose of the committee is to develop a plan for meeting client needs during major catastrophes or inclement weather. What type of plan are you developing?

   Contingency: As contingency plans are developed for problems that arise within organizations, emphasis is placed on identification of specific factors necessary to get the job done. In this case, the committee was formed for this specific task.

2. The hospital has noticed on client satisfaction surveys that clients do not feel that their pain is being adequately addressed and attended to during their hospital stay. As the quality improvement nurse, you have been asked to implement "pain" as the fifth vital sign on the client's chart. As you develop this project, consider each of the four phases of planning and state what you might do during each of the four phases.

   By nature of the project, the first phase of planning has been accomplished. The four phases of the planning process are: 1) project selection, 2) development of a solution plan, 3) implementation of the plan, and 4) monitoring and evaluation, or correcting the solution plan. Answers for phases two through four will depend on your individual problem/planning style.

3. A committee at the home health agency begins to work on a plan for inclement weather. What must be included in the plan? Identify the elements of the plan and some specific information related to each element applicable to this committee's purpose.

   Purpose and objectives
   Supportive data: advantages and disadvantages
   Budget and allocation of resources
   Timeline
   Strategies/interventions
   Identification of responsibilities
   Implementation
   Monitoring and evaluation
   Follow up

4. The nurses on the Oncology Unit are planning a health fair in the community for Lung Cancer Awareness Day. The budget for their portion of the fair is $3,000. They will provide registered nurses to take health histories, arrange for primary care provider presentations on the subject, and disseminate educational pamphlets to attendees. The general public will be charged $5 per person. How many paying participants will be needed to break even?

The budgetary break-even point will be reached when there are 600 participants ($5 x 600 = $3,000).

A loss will be incurred if there are < 600 participants.

A profit will be made if there are > 600 participants.

5. You are a nurse on the Medical-Oncology unit and frequently encounter ethical dilemmas associated with end-of-life issues. What quantitative tool for objective decision-making will assist you in making difficult decisions involving ethical dilemmas? Why?

Quantitative tool: decision grid. A decision grid helps the decision-maker compare/ describe all possible solutions. To create a decision grid for the scenario above, list ethical principles such as "fidelity" and "autonomy" horizontally along the top of the grid. Along the vertical axis, list different possible strategies (e.g., have a client care conference, call a meeting of the hospital ethics committee, facilitate a 1:1 meeting with the client, family, and primary oncologist.)

To the right of these strategies, use either a plus (+) or minus (-) sign to evaluate whether the strategy is feasible. In a true ethical dilemma, where the decision-maker must choose among two or more equally undesirable alternatives, adding +'s and -'s provides the decision-maker with an objective tool to make a difficult decision.

It is worth noting that one of the strategies listed in the scenario above includes calling a meeting of the hospital ethics committee. In a true ethical dilemma, decision making in groups is desirable. Including this strategy on the vertical axis of the decision grid adds validity and group accountability for difficult decisions.

6. What is the purpose of using case management?

Case management is a process designed to care for clients in a holistic manner. It includes optimizing care for the client to ensure positive outcomes; reducing the overall cost of hospitalization for the client and for the organization; reducing the client's length of stay, and promoting individual psychological and physical wellness (emphasizing client self-care where appropriate).

1. Staffing on a busy medical-surgical unit has been inadequate to address client acuity levels. Nursing administration is implementing 12-hour shifts instead of 8-hour shifts to cover busy parts of the workday. Using each of these approaches, how would the unit manager's approach in the change process differ?

   a. Power-coercive strategy

      This strategy is based on fear and often employs sanctions for noncompliance or rewards for compliance. In this case, the manager would inform the nursing staff the change is forthcoming and explain how it will be implemented. Those who cannot or will not adapt to the change will be fired (a rather drastic consequence, but it serves as a good example).

   b. Empirical-rational strategy

      Assumes that change will be accepted when the benefits are known and will correlate with the interest(s) of those affected. In changing to 12-hour shifts, the manager would educate the staff on the desirability of longer shifts and how working conditions will be positively affected (e.g., increased continuity of care, more teaching time).

   c. Normative-reeducative strategy

      Suggests that change will take place only after attitudes or values have changed. Self-interest and knowledge are not sufficient to bring about change as assumed by the empirical-rational strategy. The manager in this example would present the concept of 12-hour shifts to staff by asking for their reactions and inviting the group to participate in the change process. The final change may be modified to accommodate the concerns and lifestyle conflicts imposed by 12-hour shifts.

2. The nursing unit where you work is changing to a different intravenous infusion pump.

   a. Identify some specific activities that should occur during the "unfreezing" phase of this change.

      The unit manager needs to get as many of the staff members as possible to "buy-in" to the change as possible, and elicit their support in helping convince others of the benefits. Specifically, during the unfreezing phase of the change process the primary objective is to sort of "stir things up." In other words, to create discontent with the current situation. One way for the unit manager to make this happen is to continue talking about the disadvantages of the old pump and the advantages of the new one.

b. Discuss what needs to happen to enable change as you examine the possible driving and restraining forces.

In this case, some of the driving forces might be lower cost, easier to use, inadequacy of the old pump, or perhaps the old pump isn't even being manufactured anymore. Possible restraining forces might include resistance to training, sensory overload with other new policies and/or procedures, and comfort with present IV pump. Reducing the restraining forces that push against change is generally easier than increasing the driving forces, but steps in the "unfreezing" phase can involve either. Therefore, to enable this shift, initial steps should be taken to "unfreeze" attitudes about the change and reinforce the driving forces (e.g., how the new pump saves time). Find out from those resisting what their reasons are for opposing the change.

3. You are responsible for implementing a change in documentation on your unit by introducing a new system for documentation of nursing activities. You know that many staff members have complained that this will just add more work, and it is just another example of making a useless change. The staff has felt overworked all year and its members see it as more work. Would you describe the staff response as a "driving" or "restraining" force for change? What might you do to increase success with the change?

The staff response is a restraining force. A staff who feels overburdened and fatigued is typically more resistant to change. Additionally, when the staff fails to understand the benefit of the new documentation system, particularly if additional time and effort is required to learn it, their resistance to change is likely to escalate. If the members do not believe the change is important, implementation of the new system is likely to be difficult.

To increase success:

- Provide time for the staff members to discuss their reactions to the new flow sheet.
- Use their feedback.
- Explain the reasons for change and identify benefits.
- Allow staff members to participate in deciding how it will be implemented and evaluated.
- Identify reasons for staff members feeling overworked and try to resolve some of the problems identified.
- Provide time for staff members to vent in a controlled environment and then involve them in planning.

1. You have decided to accept a new position as charge nurse on a pediatric unit at a small rural hospital. Discuss the type of control you will have based on the organizational chart below.

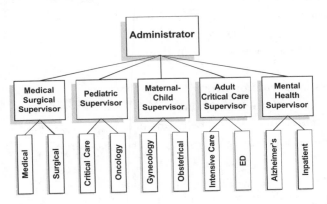

The organizational chart illustrates a flat, or decentralized structure. This means that there are fewer levels of authority and a broader span of control. For the charge nurse on the pediatric unit, this means greater decision-making ability and clearer communication since there is a shorter distance from the bottom to the top of the organization. The manager in a more decentralized organization can rely on individuals to make independent decisions. Communication patterns are simplified. There is less chance of distortion. The charge nurse may, however, need to spend more time educating other staff on effective decision-making and problem solving.

2. Think of some questions you might ask to assess the organizational culture of the institution that you are considering as a place of employment.

   a. Questions to consider asking might fall into several categories:
      - How does the organization view the physical environment and safety?
      - Is there evidence of proper and ongoing maintenance?
      - Are unit work areas and nursing stations noisy and overcrowded?
      - Is there sufficient space for private conferences?
      - Are parking lots well lit, and are security guards on duty?

b. What is the organizational power and communication structure?

- Which departments hold the most power and which are viewed as powerless?
- Who gets special parking places and beepers?
- Who has the largest office?
- Who is always addressed by their professional title or proper name?
- Is there informal communication (e.g., active grapevine)?
- How supportive is the organization?
- Is tuition reimbursement available?
- Are there comfortable employee lounges on each unit?
- Is time given to staff to attend workshops?
- Are healthy, affordable meals provided for all employees?

c. What is the organization's social environment?

- Do employees generally seem to like one another?
- Are there friendly relationships between departments?
- Does the organization host holiday gatherings or other celebrations?

3. As the nurse manager you are responsible for ordering supplies for the unit such as paper, pens, etc., as well as client supplies. You have decided to delegate this responsibility to one of the unit secretaries. The secretary has decided to enlist the help of the morning charge nurse when ordering client supplies since the unit secretary is not completely familiar with client needs. Would you consider this process of delegation and spread of authority an example of a decentralized or centralized organization?

Decentralized: A decentralized approach gives responsibility to the unit and its staff. In this example, the manager appropriately allows staff members to collaborate to find solutions to problems, instead of micromanaging every task or responsibility.

4. Compare and contrast organizational structure and process.

Key information to include:

Structure includes the components of the organization and how they are organized. Organizational charts describe the formal structure. Issues that are important are line authority, vertical and horizontal relationships, staff authority, and centralized and decentralized approaches.

Process focuses on how the organization operates. Issues that are important are communication, policies and procedures, performance, quality improvement, budget, and future plans.

1. Identify the factors affecting health care delivery in your community and the effects they have. Be specific by identifying factors and effects.

   This question requires that you discuss your own community. Consider such factors and effects as managed care, the uninsured, health care costs, changes in demographics, etc.

2. How have changes in not-for-profit health care affected the delivery of health care in the U.S.?

   Fewer hospitals are non-profit. Historically, we expect hospitals to provide care to those who have needs, regardless of their ability to pay, but this is no longer a realistic expectation. Non-profit hospitals must still make a profit to survive, but this profit is not used to pay stockholders, as it is with for-profit hospitals.

3. What is the significance of redesigning the work force and why is it important to consider right-sizing when redesigning is done?

   Redesigning the work force involves how work is done and who does it. Nurses have been affected, as their jobs have changed and many are providing less direct care.

   Right-sizing effects the number of people who are working; it typically decreases the number. As an organization analyzes how work is done and who does it, the organization must also consider the number of staff required to get the work done. Predicting those numbers is not easy.

4. You have recently become nurse manager for a medical unit. You have been told one of the goals of the unit is to decrease the operating budget. What cost-containment methods might you use?

   Some examples are to decrease overtime, assess sick time, evaluate use of supplies, institute interventions to decrease inappropriate use of supplies, assess and maintain productivity, assess employee accidents (if high, intervene to prevent), assess the use of the acuity of clients and staffing levels, assess organization of work and determine if changes are needed. Ask for staff input for cost containment.

5. What is the major difference between retrospective and prospective reimbursement, and how might each affect the hospital's or clinic's budget?

> **Retrospective reimbursement pays for services after they are provided; and prospective payment establishes payment levels before service is given. There is more incentive to control costs with prospective payment.**

6. What is a potential problem that can occur under managed care? Consider the key elements of managed care organizations.

> **Health care (who received it, type of care received, and who provides it) is controlled by managed care organizations, not by health care providers, in terms of when and how long it is provided.**

7. You work in a clinic, and you are orienting a new nurse to ambulatory care. How would you describe the role of the primary care provider to the new nurse?

> **The primary care provider is the first provider the client sees; it may be a physician or an advanced practice nurse (or physician's assistant). The PCP coordinates the client's care, and determines medical necessity, efficiency, and appropriateness of care. Referrals to specialists are done through the PCP.**

8. Select a unit that you have worked on, either as an employee or as a student. Describe the nursing care delivery system used on the unit.

> **If the information about nursing care delivery systems in this module applies to the unit you are describing, use it in your description. Try to be specific about how nursing care delivery is organized on the unit.**

9. Are the critical competencies required for a nurse who works for an MCO or for a health care organization affected by managed care any different than the competencies required for all nurses? Support your answer.

> **The critical competencies for nurses who work for an MCO or for other types of health care organizations are not really any different since nurses who work in other types of health care organizations care for clients whose care is reimbursed by MCOs. The critical competencies are critical thinking, collaboration, communication, coordination, negotiation, leadership, delegation, evaluation, and entrepreneurship. The difference might be seen in how these competencies are applied to nurse function. For example, functions such as provider liaison, benefits interpreter, and triage coordinator may require more intensive use of negotiation techniques in order to get the client's needs met.**

1. Study the nursing care delivery structure below.

   a. Discuss which type of delivery system it represents.

      The illustration represents team nursing where teams of nursing staff are formed under the direction of an experienced registered nurse (team leader). The team might be composed of another RN, a licensed practical nurse, and a nursing assistant.

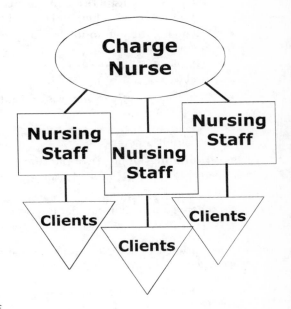

   b. What is the role of the individual at the top of the structure?

      The team leader is responsible for knowing the condition and needs of all the clients, but exact duties may vary depending on workload.

   c. What kind of leadership does this method of delivering nursing care suggest?

      Team nursing is generally associated with a democratic style of leadership. Members of the group are given as much autonomy as possible when performing assigned tasks.

   d. Discuss the issues of responsibility and accountability as they relate to this method of care delivery.

      Team members share the ultimate responsibility and accountability for care according to each job description and scope of practice.

   e. List several advantages and disadvantages of this system.

      The need for self-discipline and excellent communication skills on the part of all team members is essential in team nursing and may be difficult to accomplish. If communication is ineffective, lines of responsibility become blurred, and errors and fragmented care result. The team leader must be an excellent practitioner and leader. On a positive note, team nursing allows each person to contribute his or her own talents and skills.

2. You have just been hired as the unit manager for a long-term care facility where the morale of the nursing staff is very low and peer support is virtually nonexistent. Using your knowledge of group dynamics, think of some specific activities that could be initiated to facilitate group participation and teamwork.

> Some helpful strategies for team building include:
> - Establishing trust. Trust building begins with providing adequate information for the team to make decisions and control their work. Security is an important component.
> - Involving the staff in solving the problem; people respond best when they feel included and valued.
> - Asking all members of the nursing staff for ideas about how to solve the morale problem.
> - Listen attentively to all ideas brought forth and consider all input in the decision-making process.
> - Celebrating successes and helping build a sense of belonging by recognizing individual accomplishments.
> - Instituting 'Employee of the Month' recognition or a similar merit program.
> - Trying new ways to improve both written and verbal communication.
> - Establish a team identity. One way of doing this might be to have the nursing staff choose a new uniform that is unique to their unit.

3. The Chief Nursing Officer (CNO) in the hospital where you work has supported the team nursing model of client care delivery, but abruptly changed to the functional model of care delivery.

a. What is the most likely reason for the CNO to abruptly change the client care delivery system?

> The most likely reason is a crisis. Functional delivery of care involves task-oriented approaches to routine nursing care (vital signs and medication administration). In times of crisis, a nursing administrator may abruptly change the delivery model to meet the needs of the organization. When the crisis subsides, the organization returns to a shared delivery structure, such as team nursing.

b. What are some of the root causes of crises?

> Internal disaster
> External disaster
> Sudden turnover of nursing staff
> An epidemic

1. Why is it essential to consider goals and objectives when developing a unit budget?

> A budget is the plan for how the organization will spend the money it makes. The end is not the budget, but ensuring that the organization's goals and objectives are met. The budget needs to correlate with these goals and objectives, which give direction to the budget.

2. Explain the nurse manager's role during each phase of the budgetary process.

> Plan: Focus on the goals and objectives and set priorities.

> Develop the budget, collecting and analyzing data from past budgets, allocate resources based on priorities, and approve the budget.

> Implement and monitor the budget with analysis of variances and adjustments as needed.

3. Compare fee-for-service compensation with capitation.

> Fee-for-service compensation is the traditional compensation method in which the provider charges for services provided and the insurer pays. Capitation pays a provider to cover specific benefits for members of an insurer or MCO even if the member does not need the services. The provider keeps payment that is not used to cover services provided.

4. As a director of nursing, you are reviewing your home health agency's budget reports. What reports would you review and why?

> Budget variance report: what has been spent and the revenues. This is critical to review to determine if the budget is on target. When expense exceeds a designated percentage, explanation is needed.

> Productivity report: data about number of staff hours, number of home visits, which staff members made visits, length of these visits

> Supply variance report: supplies used, appropriateness, number compared with projected amounts

5. What is the difference between effectiveness and efficiency?

Effectiveness is doing the right things to meet the goals and objectives of the organization. Examples include evaluation of nursing care provided, and implementation of data from external reviews, for example, from the Joint Commission on Accreditation of Health Care Organizations (JCAHO).

Efficiency is doing the right things correctly. It is a combination of effectiveness and economical use of resources. It serves to meet the organization's goals in the best and least expensive ways.

6. As you consider productivity for a hospital unit, what are three examples of outputs that would be important to review?

- **Number of admissions**
- **Number of treatments (specify)**
- **Total number of client days**

7. If you have (a) some staff members who works the 8-hour shifts, based on a five-day workweek, (b) some who work evenings and nights in the same pay period, and (c) others who work the 12- hour shifts based on a three-day workweek, what types of scheduling do these staff members have?

- **Permanent**
- **Alternating/rotating shifts**
- **Flex-time**

Critical Thinking Exercise: CHAPTER 8

Human Resource Management Answer Key

1. As a team leader, you focus on the following needs of your team members. What motivation theory would apply to each of these approaches?

    a. People need to work.

    McGregor's Theory Y supports that people enjoy work and find it rewarding. When managers promote positive feedback and participation in the workplace, employees will be more creative and find greater enjoyment from their work.

    b. Self-actualization is the highest need.

    Maslow's Hierarchy of Needs. According to Maslow, success in the workplace is based on hierarchical needs, beginning with physiological (basic) needs and culminating in self-actualization (ideal accomplishment).

    c. You match work assignments to a staff member's need for achievement, power, and affiliation.

    McClelland's Basic Needs. According to McClelland's theory, three basic needs motivate people: achievement, power, and affiliation.

2. What criteria would you use to determine your own satisfaction with your job?

    This is a personal experience. Consider what you have learned from this module.

3. You are a nurse manager for an emergency department. One of the nurses has called in sick three times in the last pay period, which is unusual for this nurse. You are auditing the medical records and notice that this same nurse has made several important errors in the past month in her documentation. You decide that you need to speak with her, but as you leave your office you overhear this nurse in the treatment area complaining about the level of work and the awful work environment in the ER. What might this nurse be experiencing and how might you approach her about her absenteeism, errors and what you've overheard?

    Burnout is a sign of personal or work-related stress. Examples of burnout include (but are not limited to): absenteeism, impaired job satisfaction, job loss, deteriorating levels of proficiency and safety. To address these issues, the manager should begin by finding out the root cause of the problem. After doing so, the manager can offer assistance to the employee (if applicable), or refer the employee to an outside source such as a counselor or an employee assistance program.

4. What can be done to prevent other staff from experiencing discontentment with the level of work and work environment?

- **Involve staff in decision-making**
- **Support and listen to staff members**
- **Improve communication**
- **Evaluate workloads and staffing**
- **Provide support and mentorship to new graduates**
- **Provide stress management for staff**

5. Your next task that day is to review requests from your staff to attend several continuing education seminars. They are requesting paid time off for attending. What criteria might you use to evaluate the seminars?

- **Accreditation of the program**
- **Faculty biography**
- **Content and relevance to staff work**
- **Cost**
- **Convenience (travel time and expenses increase cost)**
- **Will the content be helpful to staff and the unit?**

6. It is time for performance appraisals for two nurses and one UAP working in the unit. Discuss the process you will use to complete these evaluations.

Data collection: Evaluation requires accurate data about the employee's performance. Methods that may be used to collect these data are anecdotal notes that are kept by the manager throughout the year, observation, checklists and rating scales, continuing education attendance records, review of medical records, incident reports, and quality improvement data.

Preparation for the performance appraisal interview: Preparation helps to make the interview more successful and a positive experience for all involved. The interviewer must be knowledgeable about the position description and relevant data about the employee, both positive and negative. The employee should come prepared with a self-evaluation and goals for the coming year.

Conducting the interview: Privacy and time are critical. There should be no interruptions. The employee may feel defensive, and the manager needs to set a tone for an open discussion. The interview needs to be documented, and the employee should be given a copy of the evaluation that is placed in the employee's personnel file.

Follow-up: The manager needs to follow-up with the employee. How is the employee doing? Are goals set during the evaluation met? If not, how can the manager assist the employee? In addition, the manager must complete organizational forms, such as forms for promotion, pay changes, etc.

7. Effective mentoring of women has become more prevalent in the workforce over the past 20 years.

   a. As a novice nurse, what are the advantages of being mentored by an experienced nurse?

   Access to information: Experienced nurses familiar with the processes and flow of information in the organization serve as effective role models.

   Power: Experienced nurses are autonomous, assertive and competent practitioners and can serve as excellent examples.

   Career opportunities: Experienced nurses can share experiences with novice nurses and assist them with career-related decision making.

   b. What are the characteristics of effective nurse mentoring?

   Mentoring is a teaching/learning process for the mentor/mentee.

   Mentoring is a reciprocal relationship.

   A gap of knowledge/competence exists between the mentor and mentee.

   The relationship between the mentor and mentee focuses on career development.

   The relationship occurs over many years.

   Mentees will eventually become mentors to other nurses.

1. What time management issues do you have?

> **Personal opinion response, but consider what you have learned in this module. For example:**
>> "My biggest time management problem is simply starting a project. I find less important things to do, putting off what I should really be doing. Once I get started on a task, I usually don't have a problem completing it—though I do get distracted by my surroundings."
>>
>> "My time management problem is knowing how many and what kind of priorities to set. I'm concerned that as I start my nursing career, that there will be so many things to remember, that I'll forget. I know this would reflect negatively on my performance, but it's really only because I'm so new at the job."

2. How might you resolve these problems?

> **Personal opinion response, but consider what you have learned in this module. For example:**
>> "The most effective way for me to resolve my problems would be to create a 'to-do' list. I should be careful that creating this list does not occupy more time than it should. Including tasks that will take a short time to complete, as well as lengthy projects is important so that I don't feel weighed down by the large things that need to be completed. Having a visual reminder of the things I need to accomplish should help to minimize distractions and keep me more task-oriented."

1. Name three reasons why it might be important for you as a manager to delegate some of your responsibilities. What three tasks do you think you could delegate and why?

> **You cannot do everything yourself. You have to find ways to get the work done, and this can happen with delegation. Delegation can improve effectiveness and efficiency of practice and thus affect productivity. Job satisfaction results from achievement of a goal. Examples of tasks that the RN can delegate include: ambulation of clients, serving diet trays and simple dressing changes. More complex tasks that can be delegated to licensed practical nurses (if within the appropriate scope of practice for that state and trained appropriately) include: care for the client on a ventilator, phlebotomy, and IV insertion.**

2. It is important to know yourself when you delegate. Take this time to honestly evaluate yourself and your use of delegation. Consider the purposes of delegation and the problems or disadvantages of using delegation.

> **There is no right answer here, but rather the opportunity to think about yourself and delegation.**

3. You are asking an unlicensed assistive personnel (UAP) on the unit to assist you in the admission process for preoperative care. What factors would you consider as you delegate this task?

> **Education and experience of the delegate, position description, time required, information that is necessary for the delegate to be successful**

> **Complexity of the task: While the RN has ultimate responsibility for completion of certain tasks, a procedure such as a complex dressing change shouldn't be delegated as it involves greater complexity than an UAP will have had experience with.**

> **Potential for harm**

> **Need for problem-solving skills**

> **Interpersonal style and communication**

> **Skills regarding carrying out the task**

1. Compare and contrast organizational structure, process, and outcomes as they apply to quality.

   Structure, process, and outcomes are used in the assessment of quality care. It is difficult to define quality. These three aspects of care provide some criteria. Structure focuses on what needs to be done in order to provide care. Process focuses on how care should be provided. Outcomes focuses on the outcomes of care, the most difficult to assess.

2. What is a clinical pathway?

   A clinical pathway is a systematic description and map of care for a specific health- related problem. Clinical pathways may describe the entire client process or a single episode of care.

3. If you work in the Utilization Review department, what types of data might you collect?

   **Reasons for admissions to treatment
   Length of stay
   Treatment course
   Discharge plans**

4. What is your opinion of health care accreditation?

   This response is a personal opinion, but consider what you have learned about accreditation.

5. Give an example of applying research findings in nurse practice (evidence-based practice).

   This response can be any finding based on research evidence. Consider what you have read in the literature and what protocols have been changed in your health care agency based on research findings. Putting this evidence in practice is an example of evidence- based practice.

Situation: You are caring for M. J., who has terminal lung cancer and is receiving hospice care. He is 45 years old, married, and has two children, ages 5 and 7. He has smoked since he was 17 and continues to smoke. His father died of lung cancer. His wife tells you that M. J. has always been concerned about his appearance. Due to chemotherapy, he has lost weight as well as his hair.

1. Based on these facts and on what you know about cancer, discuss how moral principles and values might affect your care of M.J.

Autonomy: Applying the principle of autonomy to the care of this client means the nurse respects his right to make informed decisions. This might mean for example, that the nurse respects his decision to discontinue chemotherapy even though this decision is in opposition to the nurse's personal beliefs and values.

Nonmaleficence: The principle of "Do No Harm" is especially relevant in this case since chemotherapeutic agents often have harmful side effects. Although meant to be helpful, chemotherapy drugs can do harm. Nursing care must include adequate information so that the client and significant others can make decisions based on all possible outcomes.

Fidelity: Keeping promises is applicable to every client care situation. For example, if the nurse tells the client that he/she will return to his room and check on him in 15 minutes, then every effort should be made to do so. Likewise, if the nurse assures M.J. that every effort will be made to attend to grooming measures that disguise his hair and weight loss, then a plan should be clearly placed in the client's care plan to communicate this important intervention.

Justice: Applying justice to this case is a good example of the kind of ethical dilemmas certain situations create. For instance, when thinking about equitable and fair distribution of treatment, the question becomes "Why continue administering chemotherapy to a client with lung cancer who continues to smoke?"

In addition to the moral principles discusses above, the individual values that nurses have (such as human dignity) impact client care. For example, nursing care that respects this client's human dignity and worth would include such measures as promoting independence and personal control of the situation, encouraging verbalization about his appearance, and taking measures to enhance his physical appearance before interacting with his young children. Furthermore, the nurse's commitment to caring means that the client receives quality care despite possible personal feelings about smoking and unhealthy behavior.

Situation: Mrs. P. has a history of osteoporosis. She fell in her home, sustaining a compound fracture of her left hip. She was admitted to the hospital for surgical hip repair. Her husband is extremely anxious about his wife's condition. On returning Mrs. P. from the recovery room, the transport attendant inadvertently left the chart in her room. Later, the RN found Mr. P. seated at his wife's bedside, reading the chart.

2. What ethical principle was violated?

The ethical principle of maintaining client confidentiality was violated. The transport attendant should have taken the chart to the nurse's station desk. The chart (medical record) is a legal document.

3. How would you manage this situation as the RN caring for Mrs. P.?

The RN caring for Mrs. P. should tell Mr. P. that the chart was a legal document and that he would need his wife's permission in writing to read it. Because the couple are lay persons and might not understand medical terminology, the RN should ask if they have questions and take the opportunity to educate them. Finally, the RN should inform the primary care provider that the husband had read the chart, so that he might follow up to see if the couple had other questions.

1. Describe the elements of malpractice and cite an example by applying it to the elements.

> **The nurse has a professional relationship with the client that involves providing care.**

> **For example, you, the nurse, are assigned to give medications to P.L. as ordered in the medical record.**

> **The nurse failed to observe a standard of care that is usual and customary in the specific situation. For example, you give medications to P.L. without checking her nameband with the order and medication.**

> **The client sustained harm, injury, or damage as a result of the nurse's actions.**

> **For example, P.L. is given medication intended for another client.**

> **The harm must have occurred as a direct result of the nurse's failure to observe the standard, and the nurse should have known that such failure could result in harm.**

> **For example, P.L. experiences a seizure and falls and breaks her hip due to the medication she was given.**

2. When would false imprisonment apply to a medical situation?

> **You prevent a client from leaving the hospital when you do not have a doctor's order to do so.**

3. A client was scheduled for surgical removal of one of her ovaries. During the surgery, the surgeon decides the client has a problem with her uterus and removes it. The client's consent for surgery did not mention the uterus. What type of tort is the surgeon liable for under these circumstances?

> **Battery: The surgeon in this example has intentionally, and wrongfully performed an act to the client without permission.**

4. Find out if your state has a Good Samaritan law. If so, what does it cover?

> **This question requires personal research.**

5. You make a medication error by giving the wrong medication to a client. What must you complete after recognizing your error?

   Complete an incident report.

6. Should you note in the medical record the completion of this form?

   You never mention that you have completed an incident report in the client's medical record. Incident reports are used by the organization to track client care-related problems. Nurses should document what occurred and what was done to solve the problem only.

7. What is the difference between an error of omission and an error of commission?

   An error of omission is something that is not documented, though it should have been. For example, when an incorrect medication is administered to a client. An error of commission is something that is documented when it didn't occur. For example, when one client falls while ambulating, but the nurse records the incident in another client's chart.

Bibliography

American Nurses Association. (2001). *Code of ethics for nurses with interpretive statements.* Washington, DC: Author.

Assessment Technologies Institute. (2005). *ATI-PLAN: Community health/leadership* [DVD]. Overland Park, KS: Author.

Bandman, E., and Bandman, B. (2001). *Nursing ethics through the life span* (4th ed). Upper Saddle River, NJ: Prentice Hall.

Cherry, B., and Jacob, S. R. (2004). *Contemporary nursing: issues trends, and management* (3rd ed). St. Louis, MO: Mosby.

Ellis, J. R., & Hartley, C. L., & Miller C. (2004). *Managing and coordinating nursing care* (4th ed.). Philadelphia: Lippincott, Williams & Wilkins.

Finkelman, A. W. (2000). *Managed care: A nursing perspective.* Upper Saddle River, NJ: Prentice Hall.

Gahart, B.L. & Nazareno, A. R. (2004). *Intravenous medications 2005: A handbook for nurses and allied health professionals* (21st ed.). St. Louis, MO: C.V. Mosby.

Guido, G. W. (2000). *Legal and ethical issues in nursing* (3rd ed). Upper Saddle River, NJ: Prentice Hall.

Hogan, M. A. & Smith, G. B. (2003). *Mental health nursing: Reviews and rationales.* Upper Saddle River, NJ: Prentice Hall Health.

Ignatavicius, D. D., & Workman, M. L. (2002). *Medical-surgical nursing: Critical thinking for collaborative care* (4th ed.). St. Louis, MO: C. V. Mosby.

Kelly-Heidenthal, P. (2002). *Nursing leadership and management.* Clifton Park, NY: Thomson Delmar Learning

Kelly-Heidenthal, P., & Marthaler, M. T. (2004). *Delegation of nursing care.* Clifton Park, NY: Thomson Delmar Learning.

Lewis, S.M., Heitkemper, M. M., & Dirkson, S. R. (2004). *Medical-surgical nursing: Assessment and management of clinical problems* (6th ed.). St. Louis, MO: Mosby.

Marquis, B. L., and Huston, C. J., & Jorgensen-Huston, C. (2002). *Leadership roles and management functions in nursing: Theory and application* (4th ed). Philadelphia: Lippincott Williams & Wilkins.

Marriner-Tomey, A. (2004). *Guide to nursing management and leadership* (7th ed). St. Louis, MO: C. V. Mosby.

Munoz, C., & Luckmann, J. (2005). *Transcultural communication in nursing.* (2nd ed.). Clifton Park, NY: Thomson Delmar Learning.

Sullivan, E. J. (2004). *Effective leadership and management in nursing* (6th ed.). Upper Saddle River, NJ: Prentice Hall.

Tappen, R. M., Weiss, S. A., & Whitehead, D. K. (2003). *Essentials of nursing leadership and management* (3rd ed.). Philadelphia: F. A. Davis.

Yoder-Wise, P. S. (2002). *Leading and managing in nursing* (3rd ed.). St. Louis, MO: C. V. Mosby.